Viva Library in a Book

DNA EVIDENCE AND FORENSIC SCIENCE

David E. Newton

Viva Books

New Delhi | Mumbai | Chennai | Kolkata | Bangalore | Hyderabad | Kochi | Guwahati

For David Rowand,
in all regards, the best friend one could hope for,
surely worth one more time!

First Indian Edition 2010

VIVA BOOKS PRIVATE LIMITED

- 4737/23 Ansari Road, Daryaganj, New Delhi 110 002
  E-mail: vivadelhi@vivagroupindia.net, Tel. 42242200
- 76, Service Industries, Shirvane, Sector 1, Nerul, Navi Mumbai 400 706
  E-mail: vivamumbai@vivagroupindia.net, Tel. 27721273, 27721274
- Jamals Fazal Chambers, 26 Greams Road, Chennai 600 006
  E-mail: vivachennai@vivagroupindia.net, Tel. 28290304, 28294241
- B-103, Jindal Towers, 21/1A/3 Darga Road, Kolkata 700 017
  E-mail: vivakolkata@vivagroupindia.net, Tel. 22836381, 22816713
- 7, Sovereign Park Apartments, 56-58, K. R. Road, Basavanagudi, Bangalore 560 004
  E-mail: vivabangalore@vivagroupindia.net, Tel. 26607409, 26607410
- 101-102 Mughal Marc Apartments, 3-4-637 to 641, Narayanguda, Hyderabad 500 029
  E-mail: vivahyderabad@vivagroupindia.net, Tel. 27564481, 27564482
- First Floor, Beevi Towers, SRM Road, Kaloor, Kochi 682 018, Kerala
  E-mail: vivakochi@vivagroupindia.net, Tel: 0484-2403055, 2403056
- 232, GNB Road, Beside UCO Bank, Silpukhuri, Guwahati 781 003
  E-mail: vivaguwahati@vivagroupindia.net, Tel: 0361-2666386

www.vivagroupindia.com

Published by arrangement with

Facts on File, Inc.
132 West 31st Street
New York 10001
USA

ISBN 978-81-309-1293-6

Published by Vinod Vasishtha for Viva Books Private Limited, 4737/23, Ansari Road, Daryaganj, New Delhi-110 002. Printed and bound by Anand Sons, Delhi - 110092.

CONTENTS

PART III
Appendices

PART I

OVERVIEW OF THE TOPIC

CHAPTER 1

INTRODUCTION TO DNA EVIDENCE AND FORENSIC SCIENCE

Amanda was never quite sure what happened. One moment she was fast asleep. The next, she felt the stranger's hand over her mouth. He was speaking softly to her: "Don't be afraid. Don't scream. I won't hurt you." The next few minutes were terrible, though. Then, suddenly, he was gone. Amanda heard him running down the steps and exiting through the front door. It was over and he was gone. Only later she noticed the drops of blood on the pillow case. He must have cut his hand somehow. And the police officer told her they found two fingerprints on the front door. Not much to go on to identify the intruder. But it was enough.

TRACING THE CRIMINAL

A criminal always leaves something behind at the scene of a crime, some kind of evidence that connects criminal and crime. Various forms of evidence include blood, semen, fingerprints, skin, hair, pieces of clothing, and bits of DNA. The fundamental challenge for the criminologist is to connect a piece of evidence with some specific individual—the perpetrator of the crime. That challenge consists of two parts: (1) finding, collecting, analyzing, interpreting, and preserving the evidence; and (2) locating and confirming the identity of the person with whom that evidence is associated. Today, criminologists have a host of techniques by which to achieve these objectives. They include serology (the study of blood samples), toxicology (the study of poisons and drugs), document analysis (the study of letters, forms, and other written materials), toolmarks (marks found on tools), and handwriting analysis. These tools make up the arsenal of the forensic scientist. Forensic science is the application of scientific knowledge and techniques to legal issues.

Some of these forensic tools have been in use for centuries; others have been developed only recently. Two of the oldest forensic technologies are anthropometry and fingerprint analysis. Both of these techniques are based on the same assumption: In order to connect a suspect with a crime, the criminologist must find at least one specific characteristic (or set of characteristics) that match both the evidence and the suspect, but that match no other individual anywhere in the world. For example, a forensic serologist attempts to show that the blood found at the scene of a crime could have come from only one specific person and not from anyone else.

That goal is often impossible to attain. Usually the criminologist must settle for a less rigorous standard. An investigator might show, for example, that the chance of Mr. A's being the perpetrator of a crime as 1 in 100,000 or that Ms. B was the perpetrator as 1 in 10,000,000. In such cases, law enforcement officers, judges, and juries usually have to decide what level of certainty they will accept in charging or convicting a person of a crime. Making this decision often involves complex mathematical calculations that show the probability of exclusion (the mathematical probability that a person does or does not match the available evidence), the likelihood ratio (a comparison of the probability that a person is or is not associated with a crime), or similar measures.

ANTHROPOMETRY

Anthropometry—the measurement of the size and proportions of the human body—and fingerprint analysis were developed at about the same time in the second half of the 19th century. For nearly half a century forensic scientists in various parts of the world used one or the other (and sometimes both) techniques as a way of identifying criminals. Both sciences had their adherents who declared the superiority of one method of identification or the other. Eventually fingerprinting won out within the forensic science community, although anthropometry remains an important field of study today for applications unrelated to criminology.

Anthropometry arose in the 1880s in response to an important ongoing problem in criminology: recidivism, the tendency of a person to commit crimes repeatedly. The terms "career criminal" and "repeat offender" are sometimes used today to describe recidivists. Law enforcement officers in the late 19th century held different views about recidivists and "occasional criminals," individuals who may have been involved in only one offense or a small number of crimes. They regarded recidivists as a far more serious problem that needed to be dealt with by the criminal justice system more severely to bring their career of crime to an end. (Even today, the law continues to differentiate between repeat offenders and one-time or first-time offenders in terms of sentencing and punishment. The former tend to receive longer sentences, while the latter may receive no more than warnings or mild sentences.)

The problem for law enforcement officials at the time was that recidivists were often difficult to identify. A person might change one's name, the color of his or her hair, the manner of walking and speaking, and other traits in order to hide his or her true identity. An arresting officer or magistrate might find it difficult to decide if a person was a first-time offender or someone who had passed through the legal system under different identities on many occasions.

A possible solution to this problem was proposed in the late 1870s by the French criminologist Alphonse Bertillon, at the time a clerk in the Sûreté Nationale, the French National Police. Although he held a menial job with the Sûreté, Bertillon had an ideal background for the challenge he undertook: finding a way of obtaining a positive and reliable method for identifying individuals. He was the son of Louise-Adolphe Bertillon, one of the pioneers of modern anthropology. Anthropology is a field of research in which the principles and methods of science are used to understand human beings and their cultural institutions. Alphonse grew up in a home where luminaries in the field of anthropology, such as Lambert-Adolphe-Jacques Quételet (1796–1874) and Paul Broca (1824–80) were frequent visitors, and where he was surrounded by the tools of the anthropological trade, such as measuring tapes and calipers. Small wonder that Bertillon's two brothers both became demographers and that he himself became imbued with the belief that physical measurements were key to understanding a person's character.

Finding a career did not come easily to Bertillon, however. After completing his education, he traveled somewhat aimlessly across England and France before serving in the French army. Somewhat in despair for his son, Louis-Adolphe Bertillon finally used his influence to gain an appointment for Alphonse as a junior clerk with the Sûreté. Bertillon soon discovered that record keeping and processing criminals was boring and no challenge for his intellectual skills and interests. As a result, he began spending his free time working on a new and more efficient method for identifying and classifying individuals who passed through his office. That system involved measurements of the human body that, Bertillon believed, could be used to uniquely identify any given individual.

In some respects, Bertillon's system (which eventually became known as bertillonage) was hardly revolutionary. Law enforcement officers had always made the description of criminals an essential part of their investigations. But those descriptions were usually vague and ambiguous, relying on terms such as "normal," "medium," "tall," "heavy," "slow-footed," and "dark-skinned" that can apply to many different individuals. What made

Bertillon's system revolutionary was his decision to use very precise terminology for a number of different physical characteristics. In its final form, bertillonage made use of 11 measurements: height, stretch (distance from left shoulder to right middle finger when arm is raised), bust (length of torso from top of the head to buttocks, when seated), length of head (distance from crown to forehead), width of head (distance between temples), length of right ear, length of left foot, length of left middle finger, length of left cubit (distance from elbow to tip of middle finger), width of cheeks, and length of left little finger. Bertillon chose these 11 measurements because he believed that they were the least likely of all physical characteristics to change during a person's adult life. They are all based on bone structure, a characteristic over which a person has essentially no control.

Bertillon submitted his scheme to his boss, the prefect Louis Andrieux, on October 1, 1879. Andrieux at first ignored the plan and later ridiculed it as some sort of practical joke. In fact, nothing came of Bertillon's plan until three years later when Andrieux was replaced by a new prefect, Jean Camecasse. Under pressure from a friend of Bertillon's, Camecasse agreed to allow Bertillon to try out his plan for three months. If he was able to identify only a single career criminal during that time, Camecasse said, the police would allow an extended experiment of the system.

From October 1882 to February 1883, Bertillon worked feverishly measuring every criminal on whom he could get his hands and recording those results for future reference. Finally, within days of the end of his three-month trial period, Bertillon made the first identification of a recidivist using his system. He discovered that a recently arrested suspect was the same person who had been arrested only three months earlier. Impressed by this result, Camecasse permitted Bertillon to continue with his research on body measurements, and success came more and more quickly. Bertillon discovered another career criminal in March, six more in the following three months, 15 in the next three months, and 26 more in the next three months. The effectiveness of bertillonage had been proved without a doubt. In so doing, Bertillon made one of the most important breakthroughs in forensic science.

The Rise of Bertillonage

By 1888, Camecasse had become so impressed by Bertillon's accomplishments that he created a new division within the Sûreté, the Service de l'Identité Judiciaire (Department of Judicial Identity) with Bertillon as its head. For the first time, Bertillon had the opportunity to implement his system in all the detail he had originally imagined.

One key element in the program was training for those individuals who collected the data on which bertillonage was based. Bertillon strongly emphasized the necessity that such data be collected in a precise way so that no variations due to tester differences were possible. He wrote long and detailed instructions as to how each measurement should be made. The following directions for measuring the left foot illustrate this point. The passage is considerably abbreviated, but still shows the precision required in making a measurement:

> *The operator gives the order: "Place your left foot on the tracing," and when this is done, "Lean your body forward," then: "Put your right hand on the handle of the table," and then only does he add: "Stand on the footstool on one foot only." . . .*
>
> *Before placing the [measuring] instrument, the operator should ensure himself that the toes are well in place and particularly that the great toe does not rest sideways on the stool, which would cause a deviation in its direction, and consequently a small diminution in the length of the foot. . . .*
>
> *After having verified the natural position of the body, of the foot, and particularly of the big toes, place the caliper-rule squarely, so that the fixed branch of the instrument may be exactly applied, with a very light pressure, against the back of the subject's heel and that the inner side of the heel and the joint of the big toe touch the stem. . . .*
>
> *Bring down the movable branch gradually until it is in contact with the great toe. Exert a pressure with the* right thumb *on the first and second joints of the great toe, if there is reason to fear that the too brutal pushing of the slide has bent the toe anew or that the subject himself has voluntarily drawn up his toes. . . .*
>
> *To facilitate the recoil movement of the slide, impart to the instrument a slight trepidation by gently shaking the extremity of the graduated stem with the right hand. . . .*[1]

The procedures developed by Bertillon made it possible for investigators to collect exact data that differed dramatically in quality from the generalized descriptions traditionally available to criminologists. These data consisted not only of precise numerical measurements, but also of a "morphological vocabulary" (Bertillon's term), an exact terminology to match the procedures used. For example, he found it necessary to use more than 50 different terms to describe eye color, each with its own distinctive letter code.

Perhaps the best example of the precision with which Bertillon approached his subject was his method of describing the ear. Bertillon divided the regions of ear first into four categories: border, lobe, antitragus, and folds, each of which was then further divided into four subcategories. Finally, each of the 16 subcategories was further subdivided into three to five sub-subcategories. Bertillon believed that the shape of a person's ear was as distinctive as the fingerprints on which forensic scientists now rely for identifications. In his instruction manual on the methods of bertillonage, *Signaletic Instructions Including the Theory and Practice of Anthropometrical Identification*, Bertillon devoted 15 pages to the methods to be used for taking and recording measurements of the ear.

To simplify the handling of all these data Bertillon also invented a system of abbreviations for each measurement and observation made. These abbreviations made it possible to convert a somewhat lengthy description into an easily read shorthand that Bertillon called *abridged writing*. Thus, the English sentence "cicatrix, rectininear, of a dimension of one centimeter, oblique external, on middle second phalanx of middle finger, left side, posterior face" could be written as "cic. r. of 1b ε, ml. 2d f. M. g."[2]

Another problem attacked by Bertillon was classification of the data collected from criminals. As elegant as his system was, it would have been of little value if there were no way of accessing the data. In its first few years of operation, the Department of Judicial Identity collected data on more than 100,000 individuals. However, there was no guide to aide individuals in searching through the cards.

Bertillon's classification system placed all data cards into 11 categories corresponding to the 11 physical characteristics measured. Each category was then divided into smaller classifications, and each of those classifications into more specific categories. Eventually, each of the 100,000 plus data cards ended up in a file box along with no more than about a dozen similar cards. In this way, an investigator looking for a match with a specific individual had to search through no more than about 12 cards, rather than 100,000 cards.

When properly used, bertillonage was the most powerful identification tool ever available to law enforcement officials. In France, it was used successfully to identify at first hundreds—and not much later, thousands—of recidivists. This success was a key element in the growing movement within penology to revise and improve the philosophy and methodology of prisons. It allowed the law to focus on and develop methods of treating recidivists in contrast to one-time criminals.

Bertillonage also had a number of other benefits for law enforcement officials. For example, it made possible the transmission of data about criminals across national borders and around the world. Since these data existed in numerical and symbolic forms, they could be sent by telegraph almost anywhere.

The Decline of Bertillonage

By the early 1890s, then, law enforcement agencies in most developed nations had adopted bertillonage as the primary means of identifying criminals. The outstanding success of bertillonage as a forensic tool was, however, to be short-lived. A number of factors contributed to the decline in its popularity. One of the most important factors, ironically, was the elegance of the system itself. Bertillonage was successful because it produced precise physical descriptions of individuals. But the precision of those descriptions depended on the ability of highly trained examiners to make exact observations and measurements with reliable equipment. As bertillonage spread throughout and beyond France, however, these conditions were not always met. Bertillon himself could not, of course, train every individual who used his method. And new trainees might not feel the need—or be able—to read his instruction manual with the necessary care. Also, the best measuring equipment might not always be available or, if it were, investigators might not use it with sufficient care.

As a consequence, data collected by bertillonage over time became less reliable. And once an error had been made in measurement or observation, it was almost impossible to correct. Finally, as bertillonage spread to other countries, law enforcement officials often felt it necessary to place their own "stamp" on the procedure, perhaps adding a new feature to be measured, deleting one of Bertillon's 11 characteristics, or altering the way a measurement was conducted.

In the end, the fate of bertillonage was determined less by any (or all) of these factors than it was by the simple fact that another means of identification became available: fingerprinting. This method was far simpler and at least as accurate as bertillonage in identifying criminals. Thus, by the end of the 19th century, fingerprinting had largely replaced bertillonage in most parts of the world.

Anthropometry was not, however, dead. Some criminologists and anthropologists recognized early on the potential value of bertillonage as a research tool. They saw that the precise measurements and observations produced by anthropometry might provide a way of classifying humans. The most obvious challenge was to learn how habitual criminals differ from non-criminals, what there is that can be used to identify the "criminal type." Thus, researchers collected data from both groups and compared them with each other, always looking for clues that would allow law enforcement officials to recognize those individuals who were *likely* to be criminal offenders, whether they had actually engaged in criminal behavior or not.

Bertillon himself was dubious about the use of his methodology for this purpose. He wrote that "it would be temerarious to seek from this source [anthropometry] a moral prognosis of the individual."[3] Still, the desire to find ways of identifying criminals in advance of their committing a crime has never completely disappeared. Indeed, the practice of "profiling" used by law enforcement officials today—in which individuals with physical characteristics believed to be associated with crime, such as skin color or ethnicity—is a direct descendant of that movement.

Anthropometry was also used for other less salubrious purposes, such as the eugenics movement of the early 20th century and Nazi efforts to exterminate "undesirables" in the 1930s and 1940s. The eugenics movement was a worldwide effort to "cleanse" the human race by eliminating those individuals who were physically or mentally "unfit" by some standard. The goal was to be achieved by sterilizing anyone who fell into one of those categories, thus preventing the birth of additional "defectives." A key challenge for eugenicists was identifying the "unfit," a task admirably solved, they thought, by the discovery of "unfit types" on whom eugenics procedures could be performed. Fortunately the eugenics movement was eventually discredited, and Bertillon's philosophy disappeared from that field of research.

In its efforts to eradicate "undesirables," first from Germany and later from all of Europe, the Nazis used every means possible to identify those who fell into that category, such as Jews, gypsies, and homosexuals. One technique they adopted was anthropometry. Nazi scientists were convinced that Jews and Aryans, for example, constituted two identifiably distinct human groups with measurable physical differences. By measuring the size and shape of a person's body, they expected to identify "undesirables" who had escaped detection by other means. This use of anthropometry also disappeared with the fall of Germany in World War II.

Anthropometry does have a number of beneficial applications today, however, in fields such as nutrition; ergonomics; and tool, product, and clothing design. Nutritionists use anthropometric measurements such as weight, body fat distribution, and skin fold patterns to discover the relationship among diet, nutritional status, health, and growth. Researchers in ergonomics (the study of the relationship between the human body and the working environment) use anthropometric data to design airplane and automotive seats, desks and chairs, furniture, and other equipment to better fit various types of individuals. Designers of clothing depend on anthropometric data to mass-produce general and specialized clothing that can be worn by various categories of humans.

For a brief moment in history, Alphonse Bertillon appeared to have achieved his dream of developing a perfect system for identifying criminals. Although anthropometry eventually found a number of applications outside the field of criminology, it had largely been displaced in the early 20th century within forensic science by another, more powerful tool of identification: fingerprinting.

FINGERPRINTING

The use of fingerprints as a means of identification is a very old practice. The Chinese used inked fingerprints, for example, to authenticate marriage contracts, loan and sales agreements, and other documents at least as early as the third century B.C. Although lacking in scientific analysis, such practices at least implicitly acknowledged the concept that human fingerprints are sufficiently distinctive to permit their use as tools of individualization.

A more technical understanding of fingerprint patterns had to await the birth of modern science in the 17th century. In their studies of the human body, some researchers began to develop a more detailed and more sophisticated understanding of skin and its distinguishing features. In the 1680s, for example, the English botanist and physician Nehemiah Grew (1641–1712) studied skin patterns on the fingers and palms of the hands and discovered ridges, raised pieces of skin, and pores, tiny holes in the skin that he called "little fountains" from which sweat is released. At about the same time, the Italian physician Marcello Malpighi (1628–94) was pursuing a similar line of research. In 1686 he published a work *De externo tactus organo* (On the Outermost Organs of Touch) in which he described not only the surface features seen by Grew, but also the interior structure of the skin.

Studies like those of Grew and Malpighi were conducted entirely to improve scientific understanding of the human body. None of the researchers involved saw—or looked for—any practical application of their research, such as the use of fingerprints for identification of individuals. A century later, the German researcher J. C. Mayer took the first step in that direction when he hypothesized that ridge patterns are unique, although he failed to consider the practical implications of such a possibility. The Bohemian anatomist Jan Evangelista Purkinje (1787–1869) came even closer in the 1820s when he recognized that fingerprint patterns could be classified into nine types based on the same structures by which prints are classified today: loops, whorls, and arches. In his 1823 work *A Commentary on the Physiological Examination of the Organs of Vision and the Cutaneous System* Purkinje provided illustrations of the nine types of fingerprint patterns and encouraged his colleagues to study them further, but saw no practical use for the system.

Fingerprinting as a Means of Individualization

By the mid-19th century a number of conditions were in place that made possible the realization of fingerprint patterns as a valid and reliable means of individualization. That process began in India with the work of Sir William Herschel (1833–1917), then a junior clerk in the Indian Civil Service stationed in Junipur. Included among his responsibilities was the payment of pensions to Indian soldiers who had previously worked for the British government. That task was made difficult because clerks tended to mix up pensioners, many of whom had the same or similar names. Under the circumstances, it was not uncommon for individuals to claim their pension payment more than once or to send relatives to collect a second (or third) time.

It occurred to Herschel that one method for dealing with this problem might be to have a man leave his fingerprint to acknowledge receipt for his pension, a practice he may first have observed among Chinese traders in the area. He instituted this practice in 1858 and found that it eliminated the practice of multiple payments almost immediately. Perhaps inspired by his success, Herschel made the study of fingerprints a hobby for the rest of his life. Over the next 20 years, he continued to take and re-take the prints of pensioners and prisoners in his district as well as his own. He eventually came to the key recognition that fingerprint patterns did not change over time. He found that he could put a name to any set of prints in his huge book of "Hand Marks," no matter when they had been collected.

In 1877 he wrote to the inspector general of prisons for the state of Bengal, describing his use of fingerprints and recommending its adoption in the Indian penal system. Unimpressed, the inspector general relayed his thanks for the suggestion, but declined to use it. Two years later, Herschel returned to England.

During the same period in which Herschel was using fingerprint identifications in India, Dr. Henry Faulds (1843–1930) was engaged in a similar practice in Japan. Faulds was a Scottish physician-missionary working in Tokyo, where he learned about the ancient Japanese practice of using hand and fingerprints as identifying marks for legal documents. He became fascinated with the subject and began a scientific study that led him to conclude that fingerprints could be a valid and reliable method of individualization. In the late 1870s he had an opportunity to put his study of fingerprints to practical use. During a burglary in the vicinity of his home, the perpetrator left a clean set of fingerprints on a freshly whitewashed wall. When Faulds was consulted, he took a fingerprint impression of the suspect then in custody and found that it did not match the prints on the wall. He told the police they had the wrong man, who was subsequently released. Within a matter of days, another suspect was arrested and his prints taken. This time the two sets of prints matched and the suspect confessed.

Based on this success—and later identifications—Fauld wrote a letter to the British scientific journal *Nature* describing his experience with fingerprinting (a practice that he called dactylography). The letter, now one of the most famous documents in the history of fingerprinting, was printed in the October 28, 1880, issue of *Nature*. In it Faulds noted that "[w]hen bloody finger marks or impressions on clay, glass, etc. exist, they may lead to the scientific identification of criminals."[4]

Fauld's letter is generally recognized as the first scientific publication on the use of fingerprints for identification purposes. The letter set off a chain of events—at times acrimonious—focusing on priority in the invention of fingerprinting in the forensic sciences. Herschel read Fauld's article and followed up with a letter of his own to *Nature*, pointing out that he had used fingerprinting in India more than 20 years earlier. In turn, Faulds was enraged by Herschel's letter, convinced that he (Herschel) was trying to steal Faulds' glory. To confirm his priority, Faulds wrote to a number of scientific luminaries, including Charles Darwin, outlining his right to be recognized as the founder of forensic fingerprinting.

Probably the most important consequence of this exchange was the transmission of Fauld's correspondence by Darwin to his cousin Francis Galton. Galton seized upon the subject of fingerprinting not because of its value as a tool of individualization, but, ironically, because of its possible use in classifying humans into type categories.

Francis Galton (1822–1911) was a man of enormous intellect and wide-ranging interests. He is perhaps best known today for his advocacy of eugenics, a science of which he was a pioneer and for which he provided a name. Having seen Fauld's letter, Galton became convinced that fingerprints might provide the clue that would allow him to classify individuals as "fit" or "unfit." In his usual intense fashion, he studied every aspect of fingerprint patterns and eventually wrote one of the classics in the field, *Finger Prints*, published in 1892.

Galton's book brings together many of the fundamental principles about fingerprinting on which the technology is still based. He reaffirmed the existence of specific identifying features—called *minutiae*—such as whorls, loops, and arches, that do not change throughout a person's lifetime, or even after death, until decomposition occurs. He also calculated the likelihood of there being two different fingerprint patterns anywhere in the world, and obtained a value of 1 in 64 billion. Finally, he developed a system for classifying fingerprints based on the presence or absence of whorls, loops, and arches on each of a person's ten fingers.

Galton's research proved to be fundamental to the development of fingerprinting as a forensic tool of individualization. Ironically, that research proved, however, to be completely useless in solving the problem in which he was most interested: finding a way of classifying humans into distinct racial and ethnic categories. He collected countless numbers of fingerprints from whites, blacks, Jews, and people in other categories, hoping that fingerprint patterns would provide a clear-cut way of distinguishing these groups from each other. After all, he thought, if blacks and whites, for example, have recognizable differences in skin color, hair texture, and other physical traits because of genetic differences between groups, then ought they not also to have recognizable differences in fingerprint patterns?

In fact, his extensive research on this topic produced no confirmation of this hypothesis. Except for a slightly smaller number of arches in the fingerprints of the Jews compared to non-Jews he studied, for example, he found the number of arches, loops, whorls, and other minutiae in fingerprints to be essentially the same across all ethnic, racial, and other groups. Fingerprinting turned out to be a failure as a tool for eugenics.

Interestingly enough, however, Galton's inability to find differences among fingerprint patterns (a failure labeled as "Galton's regret" by one anthropologist)[5] did not deter many of his colleagues and successors from continuing this line of research. In 1893, for example, the French psychiatrist Charles Féré reported on studies in which he examined fingerprint patterns of mental patients and of monkeys. He found that members of both groups had a higher proportion of arches than did "normal" humans. He concluded that the presence of an arch in a fingerprint pattern represented a lower stage of evolutionary development than did a loop or a whorl.[6]

Later researchers looked for similar correlations between fingerprint patterns (the presence, absence, or predominance of arches, loops, or whorls, for example) among racial or ethnic groups, among the mentally ill, among criminals, or among other groups who should, for some (supposedly) socially beneficial reason be labeled. And, as was the case with Galton himself, an acknowledged or unacknowledged aspect of such studies was the assumption that not all groups of humans are equal. Some groups, for example, might be thought of as less evolved (less human) because they possess simpler physical traits, such as arches rather than whorled fingerprints. And, of course, once that classification had been made, those groups on the lower rungs of the evolutionary scale might be thought of as worthy of less consideration than those groups that are more highly evolved (one of the basic assumptions of eugenics).

Harvard University sociologist and criminologist Simon Cole has reviewed the fascinating history of the use of fingerprints for the classification of individuals.[7] He points out that efforts to classify individuals on the basis of their fingerprint patterns are not simply a curious artifact of long-gone history, but that such research continued throughout much of the 20th century, with the most recent study in the field having been reported as late as 1991.[8] A similar line of research survives today in the interest in racial or ethnic profiling, an effort by some law enforcement officers, scientists, politicians, and others to predict in advance an individual's likelihood of committing crimes, usually not on the basis of his or her fingerprints, but on the basis of other physical attributes, such as skin color.

FINGERPRINTING DISPLACES ANTHROPOMETRY

By the end of the 19th century, anthropometry and fingerprinting were vying with each other among law enforcement officials as to which was the more reliable method of individualization. Over time, practical experience showed that the latter was the more effective tool. One of the most famous cases influencing this decision occurred in Argentina in 1892. Only a year earlier, the Argentine police department had created a fingerprint division under the direction of officer Juan Vucetich (1858–1925). Vucetich was able to solve a murder in the small town of Neochea by matching fingerprints near the crime scene with those of the murderer, the mother of the two young victims. Before long, more and more crimes were being solved through the use of fingerprints.

Vucetich made a second contribution to the development of fingerprint technology: the development of a system for classifying prints. Somewhat different from Galton's system, Vucetich's method proved to be equally effective and serves as the basis for the fingerprint classification system used in most Spanish-speaking countries today. At about the same time, Galton's system was being revised and improved by Sir Edward Henry (1863–1956), like Herschel a member of the Indian Civil Service. Henry's system, described in his 1900 book *Classification and Use of Fingerprints*, has become the basis for the system of fingerprint classification used in most of the English-speaking world. Henry went on to become a world authority of fingerprinting and in 1901 assistant commissioner of the first fingerprinting office at New Scotland Yard.

The first decade of the 20th century saw the first widespread use of fingerprinting in criminal cases. The first criminal conviction in the United Kingdom based on fingerprints occurred in 1902; the first conviction in a murder case in the country in 1905; and the first conviction in a murder case in the United States, in 1911. During the same period, law enforcement officers in many countries began to recognize the value of fingerprinting. In the United States, the New York Civil Service Commission adopted fingerprinting as a means of identification in 1902; the New York state prison system began using fingerprinting in 1903; the Leavenworth Federal Penitentiary in Kansas and the St. Louis Police Department adopted fingerprinting in 1902; and the U.S. Army started fingerprinting all of its members in 1905 (followed by the U.S. Navy in 1907 and the U.S. Marine Corps in 1908).

Courts in many countries also began to accept fingerprinting as legitimate evidence in criminal trials. This acceptance occurred gradually on a case-by-case basis with no comprehensive study of the scientific basis for fingerprinting and its reliability as a tool of individualization. In every case, the pattern was the same. A prosecutor would offer in evidence (usually) two sets of prints: one found at the scene of a crime and one obtained from a suspect. A fingerprint expert would then testify as to a match between the two sets. Almost without exception, judges and juries then tended to accept the match as sufficient proof of the charged's guilt.

The remarkable point about the incorporation of fingerprinting into the criminal justice system was the lack of any thorough scientific review that validated the underlying assumption of the fingerprinting system, especially the contention that fingerprints are unique. A forensic authority, David Ashbaugh, has written "[i]t is difficult to comprehend that a complete scientific review of friction ridge identification has not taken place at sometime during the last hundred years. A situation seems to have developed where this science grew through default."[9] For nearly a century, this defect loomed in the shadows of fingerprinting as a forensic tool, only to come fully to light in the 1993 U.S. Supreme Court case of *Daubert v. Merrell Dow Pharmaceuticals*.

FINGERPRINT SYSTEMS

The use of fingerprints for the purpose of identification rests on two basic assumptions. First, a person's fingerprint pattern begins to develop very early in life—well before birth—and it remains unchanged even after death until decomposition of the body begins. Efforts to change one's prints—by chemical, physical, or any other means—are universally unsuccessful. Second, no two people in the world (including identical twins) have exactly the same pattern of fingerprints.

Extensive research has been carried out on the first of these assumptions and there appears to be sufficient evidence to accept the permanence of fingerprints. The second assumption is more difficult to confirm experimentally since there is no practical way of taking prints from every person in the world, or even of very large numbers of individuals. Still, in all of the time that fingerprinting has been used as a means of identification, no two sets of prints from different individuals that match exactly have been found.

Fingerprints used for identification purposes are of two types: patent and latent. Patent prints are those visible to the naked eye without enhancement of any kind. For example, a person suspected of committing a crime may be asked to have his or her fingerprints taken by a law enforcement officer. The officer rolls the person's fingers, one at a time, across an ink pad and then across a blank white card. The person's fingerprint pattern shows up clearly in ink on the card. The card can then be filed for future reference.

Fingerprints deposited on a surface in the normal course of events—on a doorknob when opening a door or on a glass when a person takes a drink of water—are typically invisible. A residue of oily secretions that corresponds to the ridges on the fingers remains on the doorknob or the glass, but that residue is not visible to the naked eye. Some method must be used, then, to visualize those latent (invisible) prints. Forensic scientists have developed a number of chemical methods for converting latent prints to visible prints. For example, a surface suspected of holding latent prints may be "dusted" with a chemical that reacts with perspiration, producing a colored precipitate that is visible to the naked eye.

A fingerprint is analyzed by looking for certain characteristic features in the print that correspond to the minutiae first observed by Galton: arches, loops, and whorls. An arch is a pattern in which one or more skin ridges extend upward at some point on the fingertip, and smooth out on either side of that point. Loops are formed when a skin ridge enters from one side of the finger, forms an arch-shaped pattern, and then exits on the same side of the finger. A whorl is a pattern in which one or more skin ridges form a circular pattern around a central point. Each of the basic fingerprint patterns can be further divided into subgroups. For example, arches can be classified as plain, radial, tented, or ulnar, depending on the precise way in which the arch is formed on the fingertip. Similarly, whorls can be subdivided into plain whorls, central pocket whorls, double loop whorls, or accidental whorls.

In its most basic form, the use of fingerprints for individualization involves the comparison of two sets of prints (for example, one from a crime scene and one from a suspect), point by point. An examiner looks for very specific points of identity between the two sets, such as a double loop whorl at exactly the same position on the left thumb print in both sets of prints. A match between two sets of prints is obtained when some number of minutiae matches is obtained. That number varies from country to country, from state to state in the United States, and, sometimes, from case to case. For example, 16 matching points are required in the United Kingdom, 12 in Australia, and various numbers of matches in different states in the United States (although the FBI usually recommends a minimum of 12 matching points).

From a practical standpoint, one of the most difficult problems in the use of fingerprinting has always been the challenge of matching fingerprints from some specific individual or some specific crime scene with other fingerprints on file with a law enforcement agency. For example, suppose that police officers investigating a crime obtain very clear prints at the scene of a crime and want to find out if those prints match any fingerprints on file in their local, state, national, or international database of fingerprints. One approach, of course, would be simply to compare the crime scene prints with all known prints on file, one at a time. Since fingerprint databases now contain tens of thousands, hundreds of thousands, or millions of fingerprints, however, this approach is not practical. It is this problem that a number of forensic scientists and law enforcement officials tried to solve in the early years of fingerprint use.

One system, developed by the British criminologist Sir Edward Henry in about 1900, illustrates the approach used to solve this problem. In Henry's system, each of a person's ten fingers is assigned a numerical value, as shown in the chart below:

	Left Hand					Right Hand				
Finger	Little	Ring	Middle	Index	Thumb	Thumb	Index	Middle	Ring	Little
Number	10	9	8	7	6	1	2	3	4	5
Value	1	1	2	2	4	16	16	8	8	4

The row labeled "Value" lists the numerical value assigned to that fingerprint provided that a whorl is present on the fingertip. If a fingertip has an arch and/or a loop but no whorl, it is assigned a value of 0 (zero).

Imagine a person, then, who has a whorl pattern on the middle finger of the left hand and on the thumb of the right hand. That person's fingerprints would be assigned a value of 2 for the middle finger of the left hand and a 16 for the thumb of the right hand. In the next step of classification, a 1 is added to each of these numbers: 2 + 1 = 3 for the left hand and 16 + 1 = 17 for the right hand. Finally, a fraction is created in which the numerator is the sum of all even-fingered values and the denominator is the sum of all odd-fingered values. In this case, the numerator would be 3 (because the middle finger of the left hand has an even value (8) and the denominator would be 17 (because the thumb of the right hand has an odd value (1). This person's fingerprints would be categorized in a bin marked 3:17, which represents the fraction obtained by this method. (Note that the expression 3:17 or 3/17 is not really a fraction in the arithmetic sense, and no calculations can be made with the number. It is used purely for classification purposes.)

A law enforcement agency's fingerprint database, then, consists of 1,024 files (the maximum number of different fractions obtainable by this system), each containing all prints having the designation 1:1, 1:2, 2:1, 1:5, 7:3, 13:16, and so on. When one wishes to compare an unknown print against all available prints in the database, it is necessary to look in only one of 1,024 files for a possible match. The task may still be time-consuming, but it is about 1/1,000 as difficult without any system at all.

The Henry system of classifying fingerprints was used throughout much of the English-speaking world well into the 1990s. (A similar system developed by the Argentinian law enforcement officer Juan Vucetich has been used in the Spanish-speaking world.) It was then replaced by automated systems for classifying fingerprints. It is obvious that even with the Henry system, searching for a match between two sets of prints could be very time-consuming. But the development of the modern computer provided an obvious way of simplifying such searches. Computers are capable of examining all of the many details of a person's fingerprints, creating a permanent record of those prints (similar to the inked card traditionally used), and then comparing any two sets of prints at many times the speed of which a human is capable.

As early as the 1960s, the U.S. Federal Bureau of Investigation (FBI) had begun to explore the possibility of computerizing all of its fingerprint records and to develop a system for collecting; storing, and comparing such records. The system developed by the FBI was called the Integrated Automated Fingerprint Identification System (IAFIS), a program that was to revolutionize virtually every phase of fingerprint analysis. For example, researchers developed the Automated Fingerprint Reader System (AFRS), which uses an electronic scanner (rather than ink and fingerprint cards) to obtain a fingerprint image and then searches for matches in the FBI's database of fingerprints. A second element of IAFIS is the FBI's Electronic Fingerprint Transmission Specifications (EFTS), which permits fingerprint examiners anywhere in the world to transmit prints to FBI laboratories for analysis and comparison. With programs such as AFRS and EFTS, IAFIS has made possible a virtually unfettered exchange of fingerprint information among state, local, and federal agencies. Today, the FBI has a collection of more than 65 million fingerprints stored in IAFIS.

Legal Issues Related to the Use of Fingerprinting

The looming issue of the scientific basis of fingerprinting finally came to the forefront in the early 1990s in the case of *Daubert v. Merrell Dow Pharmaceuticals* heard by the U.S. Supreme Court on March 30, 1993. One of the questions raised in *Daubert* was what it was that constitutes "scientific evidence" in a U.S. court of law. Prior to *Daubert* the answer to that question rested on a Supreme Court decision made in 1923 in the case of *Frye v. United States*. In that decision, the Court ruled that any facts, principles, or methodologies "generally accepted" by the scientific community were admissible. In *Daubert* the Court decided that the *Frye* standard was too vague and established a set of guidelines for determining the reliability of scientific evidence. Before testimony could be entered, the Court ruled, a series of questions had to be answered:

1. Has the scientific theory or technique been empirically tested?
2. Has the scientific theory or technique been subjected to peer review and publication?
3. What is the known or potential rate of error?
4. Do standards for controlling the use of the scientific technique exist and are they maintained?
5. Is there general acceptance of the technique by the scientific community?[10]

As a result of the Court's decision, trials in which scientific evidence is to be presented may now be preceded by a so-called *Daubert* hearing, in which prosecution and defense each presents its arguments as to which evidence should be admissible and, based on the questions above, why the evidence does or does not qualify. *Daubert* hearings have introduced a new element in trials in which fingerprint evidence is an important factor. Many defense attorneys have begun to include a challenge to such evidence as part of their cases. The first challenge to fingerprint evidence occurred in *United States v. Bryon Mitchell*. In this case Mitchell was accused of being an accessory in a robbery based on his having driven the getaway car used during the crime. A match of his fingerprints with fingerprints found on the car was a key element in the case.

The defense raised a number of objections to the fingerprint evidence presented during the *Daubert* hearing preceding the case, namely that (1) fingerprint testing has not been adequately tested; (2) the rate of error in fingerprint testing is unknown; (3) no uniform standards for fingerprint analysis exist; (4) the statistical reliability of fingerprint testing has not been determined; (5) the scientific literature on fingerprinting confirms the first four points offered here; and (6) based on *Daubert* standards, courts have begun to question the validity of other forensic techniques. The defense also asked leave to call three well-known fingerprint experts who were prepared to testify that fingerprinting has not been scientifically confirmed.

The court rejected all of the defense arguments and refused to permit the testimony of its expert witnesses. Mitchell was subsequently convicted. Since that case was decided, there have been more than 40 challenges to the use of fingerprint evidence. In only one case was a challenge upheld. On January 7, 2002, Judge Louis H. Pollak in the U.S. District Court for the District of Eastern Pennsylvania, ruled that fingerprint evidence was unreliable and could not be submitted in the case of *United States v. Plaza, Costa, and Rodriguez* that he was hearing. Two months later, Judge Pollak changed his mind and agreed to permit fingerprint evidence in the case.

The future of *Daubert*-based challenges to fingerprint evidence is unclear. Questions about the reliability and validity of fingerprint evidence that were largely ignored for a century have now become the subject of vigorous debate within the legal community. Some authors have pointed out that the objections raised by the defense in *Mitchell* contain at least a kernel of truth and the continued use of fingerprinting demands that the scientific community begin studies that will definitely establish fingerprinting as a legitimate forensic tool.

On the other hand, a new forensic technique has become available with the potential for replacing fingerprinting, as fingerprinting once replaced bertillonage. That tool is DNA typing, also known as DNA fingerprinting. The scientific and legal communities have now acknowledged DNA typing as the gold standard of individualization, a methodology that confirms identity with as much certainty as is ever likely to be possible with any forensic methodology. Theoretically, then, digital fingerprinting may no longer even be needed at some time in the future. (The term *digital fingerprinting* was adopted after the discovery of DNA typing to avoid confusion between the two forms of "fingerprinting.")

The problem is that DNA typing presents a number of practical problems for law enforcement officials, including the relative difficulty in collecting evidence, greater expense, and longer delay in obtaining results. From the standpoint of ease of use alone, then, digital fingerprinting is still often the preferred method of collecting evidence. The long history of fingerprinting as a dependable tool of identification also makes a powerful argument for its continued use as one of the primary tools of forensic science for the foreseeable future.

BALLISTIC FINGERPRINTING

Digital fingerprints are only one type of evidence used by forensic analysts. Another type of evidence is ballistic fingerprints, the distinctive markings left on ammunition as a result of its use in a specific weapon. As early as the late 15th century, gunmakers found that the addition of grooves to the inner surface of a gun barrel improved the accuracy of bullets fired from the gun. They tried various numbers and types of grooves to discover a pattern that worked best. Eventually, this process, known as rifling, became standard procedure in the manufacture of weapons.

Bullets fired from rifled weapons are scratched by the grooves as they leave the gun barrel. The pattern of scratches on the bullet match those in the gun barrel. A gun barrel with seven helical grooves, for example, results in a pattern of seven helical scratches on a bullet fired from the gun. Since rifling patterns tend to differ from weapon to weapon, the patterns they produce on bullets fired from them tend to be distinctive, perhaps unique. Because of their similarity to digital fingerprints, such patterns are commonly known as ballistic fingerprints.

THE EARLY HISTORY OF BALLISTIC FINGERPRINTING

The earliest criminal case in which ballistic fingerprints were involved occurred in 1835. A Bow Street Runner (predecessors of England's Scotland Yard police force) named Henry Goddard was called in to investigate a burglary in which a butler named Randall claimed to have been involved in a gun fight with men intending to rob the house at which he worked. Goddard noticed that all of the bullets found at the scene of the crime had identical markings on them. He also discovered that a bullet mold in Randall's room contained markings that matched those in the bullets exactly. Goddard concluded that the only bullets fired at the scene came from Randall's gun. Confronted with this evidence, Randall confessed to having staged the gun battle in hopes of earning a reward from his mistress.

Three years later, a similar case took place in the United States. William Stewart, of Baltimore, Maryland, was convicted of murdering his father in order to inherit his fortune when bullets found at the crime scene were found to match those made especially for him by a local gun manufacturer.

By the end of the 19th century, criminologists had begun scientific studies of the feasibility of ballistic fingerprints as a tool of forensic science. The first classic paper on the subject was written in 1889 by the great French criminologist Alexandre Lacassagne. That paper, "La deformation des balles de revolver" (Deformation of Revolver Bullets), was published in the journal *Archive de Antropologie Criminelle et des Sciences Pénales*. It dealt with only the simplest features of rifling, the lands and grooves of which it consists. In ballistics, the term grooves refers to the milled out areas on the weapon's barrel, while lands are the flat spaces between grooves.

Over the next decade, increasingly sophisticated analyses of rifling patterns as a means of gun and weapon identification appeared in the scientific literature. One of the most influential of these papers was "The Missile and the Weapon," published in 1900 in the *Buffalo Medical Journal*. The paper was written by Dr. Albert Llewellyn Hall, sometimes called the father of firearms identification in the United States. Hall's paper considered in greater detail than had Lacassagne's the characteristic features of lands and grooves, explained how to measure rifling marks, and listed a number of important bullet and weapon characteristics, such as diameters, styles, and residues left after combustion.

Some historians of forensic science suggest that the most significant event in the early history of ballistic fingerprinting was a speech given by the French criminologist Victor Balthazard at the Congress of Legal Medicine held in Paris in May 1912. In his address, Balthazard described his part in unraveling a murder case in Tours, France, for which he had been consulted. He described the painstaking process by which he compared bullets recovered from the crime scene with a weapon owned by a suspect in the case. As a result of his studies, Balthazard found 85 distinct features in which the bullet and weapon matched, providing unassailable evidence for the suspect's guilt. Balthazard then went on to discuss the many ways in which unique matches between bullets and guns can be made, "the first time," one commentator has written, "to attempt to individualize a bullet to a weapon."[11] A year later, Balthazard compiled these findings in an article published in the *Archives of Criminal Anthropology and Legal Medicine*, establishing his right to be called the father of ballistic fingerprinting.

The Legal History of Ballistic Fingerprinting

The legitimacy of ballistic fingerprinting as evidence in a criminal trial was recognized early on in the history of criminology. For example, a state court in Minnesota called a gunsmith as an expert witness in a murder trial held in 1879. The court asked the gunsmith to examine two weapons and determine whether either could have been used in the crime being tried. The gunsmith concluded that, based on markings found on the fatal bullet and the weapons presented for his investigation, one gun could definitely be eliminated as the murder weapon, while the second might have been used. In 1902, ballistic fingerprinting (although not called by that name) was also used in a murder trial in a Massachusetts state court. Since that time, courts at all levels have been willing to consider evidence based on rifling marks on weapons and bullets as evidence in criminal cases.

The role of ballistic fingerprinting in forensic science was highlighted in the early 1920s as the result of one of the most famous criminal trials ever held in the United States. The defendants at that trial were Nicola Sacco and Bartolomeo Vanzetti, two Italian immigrants who were accused of robbing Frederick Parmenter and Alessandro Berardelli of a factory payroll valued at $15,766.51 they were carrying, and of killing the two men in the act of the robbery. After two trials, the two men were convicted of the crimes and sentenced to death. They were executed on August 23, 1927.

Ballistic fingerprinting played a critical role at the trial with both prosecution and defense offering a pair of expert witnesses to bolster their cases. Ultimately the jury chose to accept the word of prosecution witnesses in finding Sacco and Vanzetti guilty of murder. The Sacco and Vanzetti case did not die with the execution of the two men in 1927, and debates rage today about their guilt or innocence. Even 40 years after the verdict had been handed down and the two men executed, weapons used in the crime were being tested, with continued disputes as to what the results of those tests implied about the justice of the jury's decision.

The 1920s also saw the rise of the first national laboratory for the study of ballistic fingerprints, the Bureau of Forensic Ballistics, established in New York City in the early 1920s (various documents give dates ranging from 1923 to 1926 for this event). The founders of the bureau, John Fischer, Calvin H. Goddard, Charles E. Waite, and P. O. Gravelle, were all experts in the field who hoped to provide to state and local law enforcement agencies otherwise-restricted firearms identification services. Two important inventions that came out of the bureau were the comparison microscope and the helixometer. The compound microscope made it possible for an examiner to study two specimens, such as two bullets or a bullet and the bore of a gun, at the same time for the purpose of making comparisons. The helixometer was a device containing a lamp and a magnifying glass that made it possible to examine the rifling marks on the inside of a gun barrel.

Until the 1990s, the examination of bullets and weapons was carried out manually using devices such as the helixometer and comparison microscope. The process took a great deal of time and required highly trained examiners. Although useful results were often obtained, it became clear that more efficient methods for making comparisons were necessary. Thus, in the early 1990s, both the Bureau of Alcohol, Tobacco, and Firearms (ATF) and the Federal Bureau of Investigation (FBI) began to develop automated imaging systems for the comparison of weapons and bullets. The ATF's program was known as CEASEFIRE, while the FBI's system was called DRUGFIRE. The CEASEFIRE program was later reconfigured and renamed the Integrated Ballistics Imaging System (IBIS). The availability of DRUGFIRE and IBIS was only a partial solution to the problem, however. Since the ATF and FBI made use of different firearms records, federal, state, and local law enforcement agencies had to subscribe to both services, often resulting in a duplication of effort. By 1999 the two agencies decided to join forces and create a single ballistic imaging system, the National Integrated Ballistic Information Network Program (NIBIN). As of 2006, NIBIN contained more than 926,000 discrete pieces of information available to 182 state and local agencies participating in the program. In the time during which it has been in operation, NIBIN has produced more than 12,500 "hits," matches between evidence taken from crime scenes and records available in the NIBIN database. These hits provide clues that, ATF points out, are "not obtainable by other means."[12]

The Controversy over Ballistic Fingerprinting

One of the most recent events in which ballistic fingerprinting has been involved was the so-called Beltway sniper attacks that took place during October 2002. Law enforcement officials eventually arrested two men, John Allen Muhammad and Lee Boyd Malvo, for the random killings of 10 people in the Baltimore-Washington metropolitan area and along Interstate 95 in Virginia. Authorities later discovered that Muhammad and Malvo were also responsible for three murders and a series of robberies in Louisiana, Alabama, and Georgia and three additional murders in Arizona, California, and Texas.

A key element in solving this case was an analysis of ballistic markings on bullets found at the scene of the crimes and a Bushmaster .223 rifle found in the suspects' car at the time of their arrest. This evidence was critical in the conviction of Muhammad and Malvo for the crimes they had committed. It also renewed calls by a number of individuals and organizations for a national law requiring the registration of all weapons in a federal ballistics database, similar to NIBIN. One columnist for *Business Week* magazine argued that

> *Given this track record [for ballistic fingerprinting], it should now be more widely adopted by law enforcement, and it will work best if the U.S. creates a nationwide database of bullets and shell casings that could be scanned by a computer for matches with evidence found at crime scenes. Ballistic fingerprinting won't inconvenience gun owners—unless they commit a crime. Nor will it break the bank.*[13]

Other observers were less certain of the usefulness of a ballistics database. A fellow writer for *Business Week* responded in the same issue of the magazine with the observation that

> *Unfortunately, a nationwide system would probably be unworkable and needlessly expensive. Plus, it would further distract law-enforcement officers, policymakers, and voters from real-life solutions—like the hard work of catching violent criminals, fully prosecuting them under existing federal gun laws, and putting them away for a long stretch in prison without parole.*[14]

The proponents of a national ballistics database have thus far not convinced very many legislators. Only two states, Maryland and New York, have adopted laws mandating ballistic fingerprinting programs. The Maryland law, passed in 2000, requires that every handgun sold, rented, or otherwise transferred within the state be test fired before being made available to a gun dealer. The shell casing from that test firing must then be placed in a sealed container, along with additional information about the weapon, and included with the gun shipped to a dealer. The dealer must then notify the state police that the gun manufacturer has complied with state law. The New York law, also passed in 2000, shortly after adoption of the Maryland statute, contains essentially the same provisions. The theory behind the two laws is that the markings on the shell casing can then be compared with bullet or shell casings found at the scene of a crime committed in the relevant state, providing law enforcement officers with clues as to the perpetrator(s) of the crime.

Supporters and opponents of ballistic fingerprinting watched the Maryland and New York laws carefully in their first few years of operation. In both states, the results were disappointing. A report issued by the Forensic Sciences Division of the Maryland State Police in September 2004, for example, concluded that

> *Continuing problems [of the system] include the failure of the MD-IBIS to provide any meaningful hits. There have been no crime investigations*

that have been enhanced or expedited through the use of MD-IBIS. Traditional methods proved to be the pathway to solution. Guns found to be used in the commission of crime again are not the ones entered into MD-IBIS. The Program has been in existence four years at a cumulative cost of $2,567,633.

The status of the sister system to MD-IBIS, the New York State Combined Ballistic Identification System (CoBIS) was reviewed. This system has compiled almost 80,000 cartridge case profiles into their database. The result, however, is the same as Maryland. There have been no hits reported by CoBIS. . . . The annual budget request for CoBIS is approximately $4 M. . . .

The bottom line of this report is that the MD-IBIS System has failed to demonstrate the "bottom line" of the 1st Report. The MD-IBIS Program, for all its good intentions, has not proven to be a time saving tool for the Firearms Examiner or an investigative enhancement to the criminal investigator. It has simply failed in the Mission and Vision concepts originally established for the Program. Fiscal resources for the MD-IBIS Program would be well spent in other Forensic Sciences Division programs, i.e., CODIS and MAFIS, proven to be of value to the law enforcement community.[15]

To some observers, the nail in the coffin of state ballistic fingerprinting laws came with a 2001 report by the Bureau of Forensic Services of the California Department of Justice. Frederic A. Tulleners, the bureau's laboratory director, did an exhaustive study of existing laws and of technical considerations in the development of ballistic databases for handgun sales. He concluded that "[a]utomated computer matching systems [for weapons] do not provide conclusive results."[16] Tulleners provided a number of technical reasons that the state of California would simply be overwhelmed by collecting, recording, and attempting to match the number of new handguns sold in the state each year.

The debate over ballistic fingerprinting is hardly over, however. Proponents continue to believe that systems can be developed that allow law enforcement officials to compare markings on guns, shells, and bullets found at crime scenes with samples stored in government databases. In its press release, "Ballistic Fingerprints Help Solve Crimes," the Brady Campaign to Prevent Gun Violence argues that

Ballistic fingerprinting has proven effective in helping catch criminals. . . .

Ballistic fingerprinting can and does work, but the current, limited system lacks one critical element—new guns are not automatically ballistic fingerprinted and added to the database. . . . To build a nationwide database, manufacturers would test fire their guns and submit a ballistic fingerprint for each gun to the centralized system. With this database in place, law enforcement

> *could better match ballistics evidence at a crime scene to a specific gun, and then trace the gun.*
>
> *We call on Congress and state legislatures to require every gun to be ballistic fingerprinted before it is sold so police would have a database for tracing crime guns. It is time to give police this important crime-solving tool.*[17]

The Brady Campaign points to a 2002 report by the Bureau of Alcohol, Tobacco, and Firearms (ATF) on fingerprinting to support its case. In that report, ATF pointed out that

> *For several years, ATF has utilized IBIS automated ballistic comparison equipment in its firearms laboratories, and has deployed it into State and local NIBIN partner agencies in order to assist them in their efforts against violent crime. Statistics on hits generated, as well as stories of crimes solved, illustrate that these agencies—and the law-abiding Americans resident in their jurisdictions—have benefited from ATF's NIBIN Program. Though no investigative tool is perfect or will be effective in every situation, the availability of an "opencase file" of many thousands of exhibits, searchable in minutes instead of the lifetimes that would be required for an entirely manual search, provides invaluable information to law enforcement authorities.*[18]

Critics of ballistic fingerprinting believe that the ineffectiveness of the technology has already been demonstrated beyond doubt. In one of the most exhaustive studies of ballistic fingerprinting, researchers at the National Center for Policy Analysis wrote in 2003 that

> *Ballistic imaging technology cannot come remotely close to fulfilling the promises that gun control advocates make. To require ballistic registration of all new guns would most likely waste massive law enforcement resources. . . . For now, ballistic imaging mandates for noncrime guns would only hinder effective law enforcement.*[19]

The arguments over ballistic fingerprinting now center on two issues: technology and scope. Experts disagree as to whether the technical means are available for comparing bullets and casings and the weapons from which they have been fired. Resolution of this debate might be possible as the technical devices available for such comparisons are improved. The underlying problem, at least in the United States, however, is the number of weapons for which such comparisons might be necessary. The California study cited above estimated that the state would have to register 107,791 new handguns each year, resulting in a database of more than a half million such weapons in a five-year period. And this number would not include long guns, such as rifles and shotguns, automatic weapons, or other types of firearms. This number led the author of the report to conclude that size alone would make ballistic fingerprinting "so large as to be impractical."[20] The same problem exists on a national scale, where hundreds of millions of weapons are thought to be in existence, on an even larger scale. Until that problem is solved, the future of ballistic fingerprinting in the United States is very much in doubt.

POLYGRAPH TESTING

A key element in nearly all criminal cases is the taking of testimony from suspects, victims, witnesses, experts, and others with knowledge about a case. Judges and juries usually base their decision to a significant degree as to a person's guilt or innocence on the testimony they hear. Fair and just decisions require that the testimony given by a person is true. The law needs to have a way of discovering, therefore, when a person is lying about the facts of a case.

Distinguishing between true and false statements has been a problem of interest to humans for thousands of years. One of the oldest written commentaries on the problem of lie detection is a translation from about 900 B.C. of an earlier Sanskrit document. That document reports that a person who is not telling the truth can be discovered because

> *He does not answer questions, or they are evasive answers; he speaks nonsense, rubs the great toe along the ground, and shivers; his face is discolored; he rubs the roots of the hair with his fingers; and he tries by every means to leave the house.*[21]

Most cultures have developed formalized methods for the detection of lying. Many such methods rely on so-called ordeals in which a person is made to perform tasks that are thought to distinguish between truth-tellers and liars. In the red-hot iron ordeal, for example, individuals are made to place their tongues on a red hot bar of iron a certain number of times. Anyone who develops a blister on the tongue is believed to be guilty of lying.

One of the most widely used ordeals in history has been the ordeal of rice chewing, or some variation thereof. In this ordeal, a person is made to chew dry rice and then asked to swallow (in some cases) or to spit out (in other cases) the chewed rice. If the person fails the test—is unable to swallow or spits out dry or bloody rice—he or she is judged to be guilty of lying. During the Middle Ages, the Roman Catholic Church adopted a similar test for determining the veracity of clergymen (though not members of the laity), substituting dry bread and/or cheese for rice. At a later date, the same ordeal was widely used in England to detect liars.

The rice-chewing ordeal is based on a common physiological response to lying: the tendency of one's saliva glands to reduce their functioning during lying (and other strong emotions), making it difficult to moisten a dry food like rice or bread. Although clearly not a scientifically dependable test of veracity, rice chewing does have at least a modest objective basis for the detection of lying.

Over time, humans discovered other physiological responses that may be associated with lying. Literary works as far back as the third century B.C. tell of changes in pulse rate as an indication of lying. Plutarch (about A.D. 46–127) writes about the physician Erasistratus's (about 300–250 B.C.) success in discovering the lies told by one Antiochus of his passion for his stepmother, the wife of Seleucus I of Syria (a lie that was detected in any case when she bore Antiochus's child). Erasistratus made his discovery by taking Antiochus's pulse both in the presence and in the absence of the queen and when she was being discussed and not discussed. He found that the sight or mention of the queen caused a noticeable increase in Antiochus's pulse rate.

By the time of the Renaissance, pulse-taking as a test of veracity was being mentioned by a number of authorities. One of the most famous examples is found in an essay by Daniel Defoe (1659/1661–1731), "An Effectual Scheme for the Immediate Preventing of Street Robberies and Suppressing all Other Disorders of the Night," written in 1730, in which the author suggests that taking a person's pulse is a simple, harmless, and effective means of detecting subterfuge.

Science Comes to the Aid of Lie Detection

Proposals such as Defoe's found no practical applications, however, until the late 19th century. The primary barrier to development of such applications was the lack of reliable devices for measuring pulse rate, respiration, and other indicators of physiological changes associated with lying. That obstacle was largely overcome during the first half of the 19th century as the result of a number of studies on methods for detecting and measuring pulse, respiration, and other physiological phenomena. The earliest of those studies was a series of experiments carried out by the English scientist and clergyman Stephen Hales (1677–1761). Hales inserted tubes into the arteries of dogs and horses that allowed him to measure blood pressure in the animals' bodies. Hales's devices were of use for research purposes only, however. They required that incisions be made into the animal's legs, much too invasive a procedure for routine use with humans. In fact, it was not until more than 150 years later that researchers finally began to develop instruments that could be used to measure human physiological changes in a safe and routine way. The first invention of this type was the plethysmograph, invented in 1895 by the Italian physiologist Angelo Mosso (1846–1910), a student and later colleague of Cesare Lombroso (1835–1910), the father of modern scientific criminology. Mosso had carried out groundbreaking research on the anatomy and physiology of the brain, aided by access to patients who had suffered diseases or injuries that exposed portions of their brains to direct observation. On one occasion, he described the dramatic effects on brain activity caused by the fear response. He was working with a young man by the name of Bertino, whose skull had been fractured, exposing a portion of his brain. During a series of experiments with Bertino, Mosso made a striking observation:

> *The reproofs and threats which I uttered to Bertino when he was hindering my experiments by moving his head or hands, the disagreeable things which I sometimes purposely said to him, were always followed by very strong pulsations; the brain-pulse became six, seven times higher than before, the blood-vessels dilated, the brain swelled and palpitated with such violence that physiologists were astonished when they saw the reproductions of the curves published in the tables of my researches on the circulation of the brain.*[22]

By the end of the 19th century, a correlation between emotions—such as fear, anger, and passion—and certain physiological responses—such as pulse rate, respiration, and blood pressure—had been clearly established. At the same time, an important cautionary point was being made by a number of observers: Such responses to emotional stimuli are not universally observed in humans. Some individuals show no physiological responses to emotional stimuli, either for inherent reasons of their distinctive physiology or because they are able to control such responses. In 1895, for example, one of Mosso's students, Frederich Kiesow, wrote that

> *It is necessary to distinguish between different types of people. Those who emotions are readily expressed, show the most distinct changes (in blood pressure and pulse), which does not appear in people of calm disposition. In the first case, practice decreases the effect. The individual differences are explainable, not alone by temperament, but also by the different occupations of each person. A mathematician will be less emotional in mental problems which are common to his profession than one not permitted to employ himself in this manner."*[23]

This point is extremely important even today. Many critics of lie detection machines refer to Kiesow's concerns that a significant number of individuals are able to give false response to polygraph testing, making this method of lie detection of dubious value in many cases.

Studies of lie detection up to the 1890s were almost exclusively designed for research purposes. Virtually no effort had been made to discover ways in which the plethysmograph or similar devices could be used in the forensic sciences. (At least part of the reason for this fact is that forensic science did not exist to any practical extent until the late 1890s.) That situation changed in 1895 when Lombroso showed how existing instruments and techniques like the plethysmograph could be adapted for testing the veracity of suspects, victims, and witnesses in criminal cases. One device he found especially useful was the hydrosphygmograph, which had been invented by one of Mosso's students, Francis Franke. The hydrosphygmograph consisted of a water-filled tube covered with a rubber membrane. The individual being tested placed his or her hand into the tank and was asked to squeeze a metal rod. The individual was then asked a series of questions about the crime being investigated. Changes in the person's pulse rate during the questioning were transferred through the water to an air-filled tube at the top of the tank, where they were recorded on a revolving drum.

All of the earliest detection devices used for research or forensic purposes were designed to measure circulatory functions: blood pressure or pulse rate. In the early 1900s, the Italian physiologist and psychologist Vittorio Benussi (1878–1927) investigated the effects of emotional stimuli on another physiological function: respiration. He focused on measurements of the time a person takes to inhale compared to the time to exhale during periods of emotional stress. He discovered that the ratio of inhalation time to exhalation time differs when a person is telling the truth compared to when he or she is lying. With Benussi's research, three of the four elements of the modern polygraph had been developed: methods for detecting changes in blood pressure, pulse rate, and respiration. The fourth element, measurement of galvanic skin response, was not added until two decades later, as described below.

Birth of the Modern Polygraph

The instrument generally recognized by historians as the first true forensic polygraph-like machine used only one of these responses: blood pressure. It was invented in 1915 by the American psychologist and attorney William Marston (1893–1947). The machine consisted of a standard sphygmomanometer (blood pressure cuff) and stethoscope, like those still used to measure blood pressure, attached to a recording device. As the subject was asked questions, his or her blood pressure was taken periodically and recorded. A committee of psychologists reviewed Marston's invention and found it to be accurate in detecting lies 97 percent of the time. Based on these results, the committee recommended that the device be used in the interrogation of suspected spies, and Marston was appointed special assistant to the secretary of war during the last years of World War I.

(Experts in lie detection emphasize that polygraphs are not really lie detection machines. Polygraphs measure a number [poly-]) of physiological functions—such as blood pressure, pulse, and respiration—associated with emotional stimuli. One may assume that changes in emotional state are also associated with lying. But other factors—nervousness, for example—may be responsible for the same physiological changes. The polygraph is, therefore, an "emotional-change-detector"; it may or may not also be a "lie detector.")

The first machine to incorporate three of the four physiological responses used in the modern polygraph (blood pressure, pulse, and respiration) was invented in 1921 by a young medical student working for the Berkeley, California, police department, John A. Larson (1892–1983). Larson had read of Marston's work and decided to construct his own detection machine. His first effort was similar to Marston's one-function device that measured blood pressure only. He later incorporated systems for measuring pulse and respiration—a true polygraph—with results that could be recorded on a revolving drum. Larson also developed a formalized system of questioning designed to reduce errors in the results obtained with his polygraph. For example, he began his interviews with simple, nonthreatening questions designed to put subjects at ease. His work highlighted the fact that effective polygraph techniques not only require dependable hardware but also reliable interviewing techniques.

The final element in the modern polygraph—a device for measuring electrical conductivity of the skin—was not added until 1938. This improvement was made by Leonarde Keeler (1904–49), then a member of the Institute for Juvenile Research in Chicago. As a high school student, Keeler had worked with Larson as a volunteer at the Berkeley Police Department. He became fascinated with polygraph testing and spent the rest of his life working on improvements in Larson's machines. In the 1930s he invented a clip containing two electrodes that could be attached to a subject's fingertips during questioning. The electrodes measured changes in the skin's electrical conductivity, yet another indication of changes in a person's emotional state.

Scientists had known since the 1780s that electrical currents flow across the human skin and through other parts of the body. Some early researchers had even suggested that those currents might change during periods of emotional stress, probably as a result of increased perspiration that may follow emotional stress. Increased perspiration makes the skin moister, allowing charges to flow more easily. Keeler was the first person, however, to incorporate measure of such changes—called the galvanic skin response, or GSR—into a polygraph. In so doing, he created the first such machine to include all four measurements—pulse, blood pressure, respiration, and galvanic skin response—that constitute the modern polygraph.

THE POLYGRAPH AS A FORENSIC TOOL

By the time Keeler had developed the four-function polygraph, the machine had already become widely popular among law enforcement officials. The case that perhaps most dramatically brought polygraph testing to public attention was the kidnapping of Charles and Anne Lindbergh's 20-month-old child in 1932. During the trial of the suspected kidnapper, Bruno Richard Hauptmann, the world's two leading authorities on polygraph testing, Marston and Keeler, both offered to test the defendant's veracity with machines they had developed. For a variety of reasons, both offers were rejected. (One reason for the rejection was the FBI director J. Edgar Hoover's strong opposition to the use of polygraphs at the time. Hoover's objection was based on an embarrassing false arrest made by the FBI arising out of an earlier flawed polygraph test.)

The Lindbergh case took place just as interest in polygraph testing was spreading through state and local law enforcement agencies in the United States. One of the last agencies to adopt polygraph testing was the FBI, largely as a result of Hoover's opposition to the technology. It was not until 1938 that the agency began using polygraph testing in espionage investigations, although not in routine domestic criminal investigations. At about the same time, one of the bureau's special agents, E. P. Coffey, established the first polygraph research program in the federal government.

The 1930s and 1940s also saw the growth of schools, organizations, journals, and other elements that make up the formal structure of a profession of polygraphy. Keeler began teaching a two-week course in the subject to law enforcement and military personnel in Chicago in 1942 and expanded the course to six weeks in 1948, establishing the first school of polygraphy—the Keeler Polygraphy Institute—in the process.

Polygraph testing remains very popular in the early 21st century for two purposes: the investigation of crimes and the screening of individuals for employment. Dozens of companies exist to provide the services of trained polygraph examiners, and 20 specialized schools in 12 U.S. states and six foreign countries exist for training specialists in the field. The nation's primary association of polygraph examiners—the American Polygraph Association—claims to have more than 3,200 members, and it sponsors an active program of training and professional support for its members.

Polygraph testing also remains an essential component of many federal programs. Agencies such as the FBI; Secret Service; Central Intelligence Agency (CIA); Drug Enforcement Administration (DEA); National Security Agency (NSA); Department of Energy (DOE); Department of Defense (DoD); Bureau of Alcohol, Tobacco and Firearms (ATF); Defense Security Service; and the U.S. Marshals Service all use polygraph testing routinely for both pre-employment and in-service purposes. There is little doubt that polygraph testing has wide and enthusiastic support in law enforcement agencies at all levels of government and among human resource departments in companies of all sizes and types.

LEGAL ISSUES ASSOCIATED WITH POLYGRAPH TESTING

This fact contrasts quite dramatically with longstanding doubts about the validity of polygraph testing as a means of discovering subterfuge. These doubts first surfaced in the earliest history of the modern polygraph. Perhaps the most famous case from that period arose out of the murder of Berkeley, California, physician Robert W. Brown in 1921. Seven months after the crime had been committed, James Frye confessed to the murder, a confession that he later recanted. In attempting to determine the truth or untruth of Frye's statements, John Larson of the Berkeley Police Department administered a test using his newly-invented "lie detector" machine. The test indicated that Frye had not murdered Brown.

When Frye was eventually tried for the Brown murder, his defense attorney attempted to offer in evidence the results of Larson's test. The trial court ruled that evidence to be inadmissible. That court's ruling was later affirmed by the Court of Appeals for the District of Columbia, which said that methods for the testing of a person's veracity—like Larson's machine—were too new to have been tested and evaluated by the scientific community and that, therefore, the scientific validity of lie detection by such means had not yet been established. It ruled that scientific evidence is admissible in a court of law only when the theory and practice on which that evidence is based has been "sufficiently established to have gained general acceptance in the particular field to which it belongs."[24] It went on to say that the results of "lie detection" tests did not yet meet that standard.

The *Frye* decision turned out to be one of immense significance in American jurisprudence. It remained the standard for deciding the admissibility of scientific evidence for more than 50 years with significance not only for cases involving polygraph testing, but also for cases involving any other type of scientific forensic tests. Throughout the long reign of the *Frye* standard, a legal precedent developed in which polygraph results were ruled admissible only when both parties to a case agreed to accept the validity of those results. The precedent was based on the fact that no court during the period was ever convinced that the basis for the *Frye* decision—acceptance by the scientific community of the validity of polygraph testing—had been met.

The *Frye* standard was eventually superceded in 1975 with the adoption of the Federal Rules of Evidence and in 1993 by the U.S. Supreme Court's decision in the case of *Daubert v. Merrell Dow*. In that case, the Court established a four-prong test for the admissibility of scientific evidence (such as that obtained by polygraph testing). A trial court had to consider the following factors in determining whether or not scientific testimony is admissible:

1. Has the scientific theory or technique been empirically tested?
2. Has the scientific theory or technique been subjected to peer review and publication?
3. What is the known or potential error rate?
4. What is the expert's qualifications and stature in the scientific community?[25]

As a consequence of this ruling, the admissibility of scientific evidence today is generally decided by a so-called *Daubert* hearing that precedes the actual court case. In the *Daubert* hearing, attorneys for prosecution and defense present evidence as to why testimony by "experts" in the field should or should not be admitted in the case that is to follow.

The U.S. Supreme Court has also spoken on the admissibility of polygraph testing results in other cases. In a 1998 case, *U.S. v. Scheffer*, the Court ruled on a lower-court decision in which the defendant, Edward Scheffer, had asked to include the results of a polygraph test that would have supported his claim of innocence in a crime for which he had been convicted. The Court decided that the scientific basis for polygraph testing had still not been established and that evidence based on such tests still did not meet the existing standards for admissibility. Writing for the Court, Justice Clarence Thomas said that "[t]he contentions of respondent and the dissent notwithstanding, there is simply no consensus that polygraph evidence is reliable."[26] The Scheffer decision remains the standard for court cases involving polygraph testing in the United States today.

Studies on Polygraph Testing

Aside from the history of court decisions on polygraph testing, the question of the scientific validity of results of such testing remains an active field of research within the scientific and legal communities. Throughout the long history of scientific lie detection, scholars have searched for concrete, verifiable correlations between verbal statements ("true statements" and "lies") and physiological phenomena such as pulse rate, blood pressure, respiration, galvanic skin response, and, more recently, responses such as voice stress analysis and brain wave fingerprinting. They have attempted to answer the question: What physical response does a subject who lies give that can be associated with 100 percent (or nearly 100 percent) certainty?

The long history of this research has been summarized not only in judicial opinions such as *United States v. Scheffer*, but also in a number of reviews by scientific academies and governmental agencies. Two of the most important of those reviews were studies conducted by the U.S. Congress Office of Technology Assessment (OTA) in 1983 and by the National Research Council (NRC) of the National Academies of Science in 2002.

The OTA study, "Scientific Validity of Polygraph Testing: A Research Review and Evaluation," included research conducted by its own staff in addition to review of 30 earlier studies and reviews. It found that the results of polygraph testing varied widely, producing accurate results anywhere from 64 to 98 percent of cases. Overall, the rate of correct guilty responses ranged from 70.6 percent to 98.6 percent, and the correct innocent responses, from 12.5 percent to 94.1 percent. The OTA study also examined the number of false positive responses (when an innocent person is thought to be providing deceptive responses) and false negative responses (when a guilty person provides deceptive responses). It found false positives in anywhere from 0 to 75 percent of cases (with an average of 19.1 percent) and the number of false negatives, from 0 to 29.4 percent (with an average of 10.2 percent). In other words, examiners on average would have misidentified an innocent person about one time out of five and a guilty person about one time out of 10.

The OTA concluded that a major problem with polygraph testing was the variation in examiners' training and skill and in conditions under which tests were carried out. It also wrote that the theory of polygraph testing still "is only partially developed and researched" and that much more additional research is needed in the fields of psychology, physiology, psychiatry, neuroscience, and medicine in order to provide an adequate scientific basis for polygraph testing.[27]

The NRC study, *The Polygraph and Lie Detection*, conducted almost 20 years later, produced strikingly similar conclusions. It undertook to review research on the use of polygraph testing in three situations: single-event testing (essentially, forensic investigations of a crime), pre-employment screening, and in-service employment screening. The NRC selected 57 studies in the first category and only one in the latter two categories. The methodology of that one study, however, was too flawed to use. The committee was forced, therefore, to rely on the 57 single-event studies and anecdotal evidence for its conclusion.

Overall, the NRC reviewers noted that modern polygraph testing is nearly a century old and that one might expect that, by this time, a consistent and valid scientific basis might have been developed. Such is apparently not the case, however. "Polygraph research has not developed and tested theories of the underlying factors that produced the observed responses," the NRC committee pointed out.[28] In addition, as the OTA had observed 20 years earlier, conditions under which polygraph testing takes place vary widely and are highly subject to human variability. That is, a variety of factors are responsible for the changes in observed physiological responses, such as blood pressure and pulse rate, guilt being only one factor. As a consequence, the NRC report predicted that further refinements in polygraph technology were likely to produce only marginal improvements in accuracy: Polygraph testing may now be as efficient in detecting lies as it will ever be.

The NRC's final conclusions were not very encouraging for proponents of polygraph testing. The committee wrote that the technology can detect lying "well above chance, though well below perfection."[29] Error is such an inherent part of polygraph testing, the committee concluded, that information gained by the procedure is always subject to significant doubt.

Proponents of polygraph testing were, of course, less than enthusiastic about the NRC's report. They found a number of reasons to question the conclusions drawn in the study. For example, in a press release produced in response to the NRC report, the American Polygraph Association (APA) pointed out that the NRC committee had relied on only 57 of more than 1,000 studies conducted on the accuracy of polygraph testing and that the association itself had not been invited to contribute to the committee's deliberations. While agreeing with many of the committee's conclusions, the APA concluded its press release by pointing out that "none of [the] alternatives [to polygraph testing] outperform, nor do any of them yet show promise of supplanting the polygraph in the near term."[30] The implication was that flawed as it may be, polygraph testing still has an important role to play in the detection of subterfuge in criminal cases and employment testing.

The Legal Status of Polygraph Testing

State and federal governments have long acknowledged and accepted the weaknesses of polygraph testing. As early as 1959, Massachusetts adopted the first state law prohibiting the use of polygraph testing in making employment decisions.[31] Other states followed the Massachusetts example, but such laws were rendered moot by passage of a federal statute, the 1988 Employee Polygraph Protection Act (EPPA). That act made it illegal for employers to require a polygraph test as a condition of employment, with exceptions for industries in certain fields, such as security, law enforcement, and certain governmental agencies. In 1991 the EPPA was extended to include the military with the adoption of Military Rule of Evidence 707, which prohibits the admission of evidence obtained by polygraph testing in any court martial.

The Current Status of Polygraph Testing in the United States

As of the early 21st century, researchers have generally been unable to demonstrate a strong scientific basis for the use of polygraph testing in lie detection. Virtually no theoretical basis for polygraphy has been developed by scholars in the field, and experimental studies tend to show significantly large error rates in the use of polygraphs for testing the truth and fallacy of statements. At least partly as a result of these studies, a number of governmental agencies have limited the use of polygraphs in determining the guilt and innocence of individuals. Most court systems also place severe restrictions on the admissibility of evidence obtained from polygraph testing. Under such circumstances, one might anticipate a reduced interest in using polygraphs for testing the guilt or innocence of individuals suspected of crimes.

Such, however, is not the case. Instead, polygraphy has become a widely popular tool for lie detection in a number of applications in the United States and, to a lesser extent, in some other countries around the world. Polygraph testing by companies for employment and pre-employment screening has diminished to a considerable extent as a result of the 1988 EPPA. However, testing by and for companies and agencies exempted from the act has in many cases expanded. The American Polygraph Association has listed a number of agencies that make use of polygraph testing, including federal and state law enforcement agencies, such as police and sheriff's departments; members of the legal community, such as U.S. attorney offices, district attorney offices, public defender offices, defense attorneys, and parole and probation departments; and individuals and organizations in the private sector, including companies and corporations (as restricted and limited by the Employee Polygraph Protection Act of 1988); private citizens dealing with matters not involving the legal or criminal justice system; and attorneys in civil litigation.

Agencies of the federal government that are exempt from the EPPA have also been especially active in the use of polygraph testing. The September 2006 "Semiannual Report to Congress" of the U.S. Department of Justice, for example, reported that federal agencies such as the Federal Bureau of Investigation (FBI); Drug Enforcement Administration (DEA); and the Bureau of Alcohol, Tobacco, and Firearms (ATF) had conducted more than 49,000 polygraph examinations in fiscal years 2002 through 2005. More than half of those examinations were pre-employment screening tests, while another 17 percent were part of criminal investigations. During the same period, the number of in-service employment screenings conducted by the FBI alone increased by 78 percent.[32]

The question has been raised on a number of occasions as to how a technology with so many apparent flaws can remain so popular as a technique for the detection of lying. As noted above, proponents argue that, whatever flaws polygraph testing may have, it produces results superior to those of any other lie detection technology. In addition, they point out that the very act of testing may elicit a confession of guilt from the subject. That is, many people probably still trust the accuracy of a polygraph, scientific evidence to the contrary notwithstanding, to believe that the truth will be uncovered in an interview in any case. So they decide simply to confess and avoid having to undergo the procedure. The status of polygraph testing is probably more complex then suggested by this simplistic answer alone. In any case, the future of polygraphy as a forensic tool for at least the near future seems secure.

DNA TYPING

One of the most fundamental challenges in forensic science is individualization: determining the identify of a person (such as the perpetrator of a crime) with a high degree of specificity. Law enforcement officials must be able to say that the person who committed a violent crime or a murder was Mr. A. or Ms. B., not the next-door neighbor, a good friend, or even a close relative. Fingerprinting has long been the most reliable method of individualization, based on the belief that no two individuals in the world have exactly the same set of fingerprint patterns. Fingerprinting poses both theoretical and practical problems, however, in that scientists have not yet proved this underlying assumption, and the collection and interpretation of fingerprints is often difficult.

In 1984, the British geneticist Alec Jeffreys (1950–) discovered a new method of individualization with the promise of its becoming the perfect method for distinguishing any two humans from each other. The method, based on small variations in the DNA of all humans, was originally called DNA fingerprinting, because of its similarity to traditional fingerprinting. The method is now more commonly called DNA typing, DNA profiling, or DNA patterning.

The acronym DNA is short for deoxyribonucleic acid, the name given to a group of molecules that occur in all cells of all living organisms and that carry that organism's genetic information. That is, they carry the instructions for making the chemical compounds—proteins—by which cells stay alive, grow, develop, reproduce, and carry out all of the functions that constitute life as we know it.

THE STRUCTURE OF DNA MOLECULES

DNA molecules are very large, complex molecules made, nonetheless, of only a few relatively simple units: a sugar called deoxyribose (D); a combination of phosphorus and oxygen atoms called a phosphate group (P); and four nitrogen bases, adenine (A), cytosine (C), guanine (G), and thymine (T). Nitrogen bases are compounds in which carbon and nitrogen atoms are joined to each other in a ring. The combination of one sugar molecule, one phosphate group, and any one nitrogen base (of the form D - P - A, for example) is called a nucleotide. A complete DNA molecule consists of very long chains of thousands of nucleotides joined to each other, as represented by the following abbreviated formula:

$$- N_1 - N_2 - N_4 - N_4 - N_1 - N_2 - N_3 -$$

where N_1, N_2, N_3, and N_4 represent the four possible types of nucleotides, each having a different nitrogen base joined to a sugar and phosphate. Each DNA molecule actually contains a pair of nucleotide chains twisted around each other, somewhat in the form of a spiral staircase, in a structure called a double helix.

When scientists describe a DNA molecule, they usually do so by listing the sequence of nitrogen bases in the molecule. The "backbone" to which the bases are attached is a repetitive sequence of the form - D - P - D - P - D - P - D - P - which provides no unique information about the molecule. Thus, one might want to talk about a specific portion of one specific DNA molecule in which the nitrogen base sequence can be described as - A - G - G - G - A - D - T - T -. If that segment of DNA carries useful genetic information—that is, if it tells a cell how to perform some function—it constitutes or is part of a gene. Genes occur in slightly different forms in organisms known as alleles. For example, the gene that tells a cell how to make hair exists in forms that carry the instructions for black hair, red hair, brown hair, or hair of some other color.

Less than one-tenth of 1 percent of the nitrogen base sequences in DNA molecules carry no genetic information, that is, they carry no known useful information for cells. Scientists call such sequences "junk DNA" or, more formally, introns. An intron is a sequence of nitrogen bases with no known human genetic function *in*terspersed between ex*on*s, nitrogen base sequences that do carry information and are, therefore, usually *ex*pressed in a cell. Although the exons in humans are all very similar to each other (most humans at birth all have two eyes, two ears, one nose, two arms, similar brains, and other structures in common with each other), their introns differ widely. Because of this wide variability, scientists can use the molecular structure of introns to distinguish between any two members of a species: between any two humans, any two killer whales, or any two English sparrows, for example.

As with fingerprinting, scientists cannot say with absolute certainty that no two humans (or two members of any species) are absolutely unique. (In fact, identical twins do share exactly the same DNA patterns.) It is possible, however, for one to calculate the likelihood that any two persons will have exactly the same sequence of nitrogen bases, the same DNA "fingerprint." Because DNA is such a large and complex molecule, those probabilities are very small indeed. In forensic cases, it is generally not difficult to say that the chance of finding a given DNA pattern in two different individuals is one in 10 million or one in 100 million, one in a billion, or some similar very low frequency. Because of this high level of certainty in identifying a specific individual based on his or her DNA, DNA typing has now replaced digital fingerprinting as the "gold standard" of individualization in forensic science.

DNA typing is superior to digital fingerprinting and other forensic techniques not only because it discriminates between two people better than any other procedure, but also because it can be used with a broader range of sample types. A digital fingerprint can be obtained only from a person's fingertips (or, less commonly, from the palms, toes, or soles of the feet). But DNA occurs in every cell of the body. All an investigator needs is a drop of blood, a single hair, a flake of skin, or a single cell from any other part of the body to obtain a DNA fingerprint. DNA typing can also be carried out with very small samples and with evidence that is months, years, decades, or even centuries old. Unlike blood and other types of evidence that degrades over time, DNA taken from a cell often remains in perfect condition for virtually unlimited periods of time.

The Early History of Forensic DNA Typing

Alec Jeffrey's great accomplishment was his discovery of a method by which scientists can find the sections of DNA that differ in individuals, snip them out of a DNA chain, and take their "photographs" using radioactive materials. The method he developed is known as restriction fragment length polymorphisms (RFLP), a name that comes from the chemical compounds used to do the snipping (restriction enzymes), the size of the segments snipped out, and the variations (polymorphisms) present in the segments. Today RFLP has largely been replaced by a second method for finding, cutting out, and identifying portions of a DNA molecule. That method, invented by American molecule biologist Kary Mullis (1944–) in 1986 is called polymerase chain reaction (PCR). Virtually all forensic applications of DNA typing now use the PCR technique because it is faster and can be used with much smaller samples of DNA than can RFLP.

Less than a year after Jeffreys discovered the RFLP method, he had an opportunity to use the technique in solving a practical problem in genetics. The problem concerned a young boy who attempted to enter the United Kingdom from Ghana with a British passport that appeared to officials to have been altered. The boy claimed that he was returning to his mother in England after a visit to Ghana. Immigration officials suspected, however, that the boy was a relative of the person named in the passport, perhaps a cousin, trying to enter the country illegally. At first, Jeffreys thought the problem was beyond the scope of science. "Well, forget it!" he said at first. "This is a jigsaw puzzle with too many pieces missing."[33]

He eventually decided to try using RFLP, however, to solve that puzzle. He took blood samples from the boy, the boy's mother, his father, and three sisters for RFLP analysis. He found the six samples were sufficiently similar that there could be no question as to the relationships claimed for the family. The boy was admitted to the United Kingdom.

About a year after the Ghanaian case was solved, Jeffreys received his first request to become involved in a criminal investigation. The case involved a pair of rape-murders in the small town of Narborough in Leicestershire, one that occurred in 1983, the other in 1986. Police had arrested a local boy named Richard Buckland for the crimes. Buckland confessed to the 1986 crime but denied any involvement in the earlier case. Leicestershire police asked Jeffreys to use his DNA test to confirm Buckland's guilt in both crimes. Jeffreys examined DNA taken from semen at both murder scenes and DNA from a sample of Buckland's blood. He confirmed that the same person had committed both rape-murders, but that Buckland was not that person. Buckland was exonerated of both crimes, the first person in history to have been found innocent as a result of DNA typing.

The Leicestershire case had a somewhat bizarre conclusion. Police eventually took blood samples from all males in Narborough and two nearby villages. Jeffreys found no match with DNA taken from the crime scene and any of the more than 400 samples collected by the police. The case appeared to be insolvable, at least by means of DNA typing. The unexpected turn came about a year later when a Narborough woman overhead a fellow worker bragging that he had given a sample of his blood under the name of a friend, Colin Pitchfork. Pitchfork was arrested and his DNA tested. It matched the samples taken from the two crime scenes, and he was convicted of the two crimes.

DNA Typing in Court Cases in the United States

The success of DNA typing in solving the Leicestershire case soon became widely known. Prosecutors in many countries recognized the power of the new technology and began to use it eagerly. As Ron Fridell has written in his book *DNA Fingerprinting: The Ultimate Identity*, "[n]ever before in the history of law enforcement had a new technique for analysis of physical evidence been adopted so suddenly and so unreservedly. It seemed as if DNA fingerprinting were foolproof."[34]

In the United States, the first laboratory established specifically to carry out DNA typing was Cellmark Diagnostics, opened in Germantown, Maryland, in 1987. Cellmark trademarked the phrase "DNA Fingerprinting" to denote the specific details of the technology it had developed for DNA typing. Cellmark's only competitor in the field of DNA typing in the United States was Lifecodes Laboratories of Valhalla, New York. Lifecodes had been founded in 1982 and began DNA testing in 1987, shortly after Cellmark began operations. Lifecodes was hired in November 1987 by prosecutors in Orange City, Florida, to test semen samples found at the scene of a rape for which Tommy Lee Andrews had been arrested. Lifecodes reported that the DNA found at the crime scene matched Andrews's DNA with a probability of one in 10 billion. (That is, the company said that the chance of there being some other person with exactly the same DNA sample was one in 10 billion.) Convinced to a large extent by the strong DNA evidence, a jury convicted Andrews of rape. He was sentenced to 22 years in prison. A year later, the Florida District Court of Appeals upheld the lower court's verdict, giving Andrews the dubious honor of being the first person in the United States to have had his or her conviction upheld by a higher court on the basis of DNA evidence.

The Andrews case was reported and commented on widely in the popular press and in legal journals, opening the floodgates to its use in a number of criminal cases. Within a year of the Andrews decision, DNA typing had also been affirmed for the first time by a highest state court, the West Virginia Supreme Court of Appeals in the case of *State v. Woodall* (385 S.E. 2d 253; W. Va. 1989). It seemed that DNA testing was on its way to general and enthusiastic acceptance within the law enforcement and legal communities.

Then came *People v. Castro*. The case arose out of the arrest of a 38-year-old Latino man, Jose Castro, for the murder of a neighbor, Vilma Ponce, and her two-year-old daughter. Mother and daughter had been stabbed to death in their apartment, and blood found on Castro's watch was thought by police to belong to one or both of the victims. Lifecodes conducted a DNA analysis of the blood sample and compared it with DNA taken from the two victims. The company reported the likelihood of finding the match produced was one in 100 million. As in previous cases, the DNA evidence was so strong that a conviction appeared certain.

At that point, however, attorneys for Castro took a step that no defense attorney had yet used: They challenged the scientific validity of the DNA analysis. The two attorneys, Barry C. Scheck and Peter J. Neufeld (who were later to found the Innocence Project, designed to exonerate individuals falsely convicted of crimes) argued that DNA typing was a new technology that had not yet been adequately tested. They based their argument on the existing standard for the admissibility of scientific evidence in a criminal trial, established 60 years earlier in *Frye v. United States*. According to the *Frye* standard, scientific evidence had to meet a number of criteria to be admissible in a criminal trial, one of which was that the procedure must have been widely accepted by the scientific community. Scheck and Neufeld argued that DNA typing had not yet reached that level of approval.

Judge Gerald Sheindlin applied the *Frye* standard to the Lifecodes DNA typing results and found that they did meet most of the standards imposed by that precedent. He wrote in his decision that the scientific community was in general agreement that DNA testing produces valid results in terms of its ability to discriminate among specific individuals. DNA typing is valid also, he said, because it makes use of techniques that were in existence even before DNA typing had been invented.

The problem in this case, however, was that Lifecodes had, purely and simply, made technical errors in carrying out DNA testing of blood samples. Not only had it made technical errors, but it had also misjudged the probability of a match between blood samples. Simply stated, company scientists had said the DNA "fingerprints" from the blood on Castro's watch and the two victims matched when they did not. The evidence provided by Lifecodes failed the final prong of the *Frye* test, then, because it was not obtained by the proper application of accepted methods. As a result, Sheindlin excluded the DNA evidence from consideration in the case. (Castro later confessed to the murders and was sentenced to life in prison.)

People v. Castro is an especially important court case because it established the general principle for the admissibility of DNA evidence. It said that the theory and technology of DNA typing is well established and widely accepted by the scientific community, producing valid results when testing is properly conducted. Other courts have confirmed and adopted this principle, and it provides the foundation on which DNA typing rests today. The other part of the Castro principle, however, is that laboratories must follow typing procedures with the greatest care in order to obtain valid results. The only question courts have to answer in considering DNA evidence is whether this part of the standard has been observed and whether testing laboratories have avoided the introduction of human error into their results (as Lifecodes failed to do in *Castro*).

The first federal case in which these standards were applied and DNA typing validated was *United States v. Jakobetz*, decided by the U.S. Court of Appeals for the Second District in 1992. The case arose when Randolph Jakobetz, a truck driver, was arrested for the violent rape of a woman he surprised and subdued at a rest stop on Interstate 91 in Westminster, Vermont. In presenting its case, the prosecution offered DNA evidence from a blood sample provided by the accused and semen taken from the woman's body. The testing laboratory determined that the probability of a match of the two samples was 1 in 300 million. Based in part on this evidence, Jakobetz was convicted of the crime. He appealed the trial court's decision, arguing that the DNA evidence submitted in the case was unreliable. His appeal was rejected by the court of appeals, a decision that the U.S. Supreme Court declined to review. The appeals court decision not only affirmed the lower court's decision, but noted that future cases should consider Jakobetz as a precedent in dealing with DNA evidence. It wrote that

> *We thus conclude that the district court properly exercised its discretion in admitting the DNA profiling evidence proffered by the government in this case; we also conclude that courts facing a similar issue in the future can take judicial notice of the general theories and specific techniques involved in DNA profiling.*[35]

THE DEBATE OVER DNA TYPING IN FORENSIC SCIENCE

By 1990, experts and interested observers had begun to take sides on the use of DNA typing as a source of valid evidence in criminal cases. On the one side were most prosecuting attorneys, law enforcement officials, scientists familiar with DNA technology, and, of course, laboratories who conducted DNA testing. These individuals were convinced that DNA typing was, as one judge put it, "the single greatest advance in the search for truth since the advent of *cross-examination* [italics in original]."[36]

On the other side were many defense lawyers, a large fraction of the media, and many ordinary citizens, many of whom were unfamiliar with DNA technology and unconvinced of the extraordinary claims being made for it. Leading spokespersons for the anti-DNA typing camp were Barry Scheck and Peter Neufeld, defense attorneys in the Castro case. They established the DNA Task Force, a committee within the National Association of Criminal Defense Lawyers to limit or prohibit the use of DNA evidence in criminal cases. The Task Force's efforts had little effect on the legal system, where judges continued to accept DNA evidence and prosecutors relied more and more on such evidence in their cases. But anti-DNA arguments were often persuasive among representatives of the media and general public who often felt the power of DNA typing was being overstated.

In 1990, the National Research Council of the National Academy of Sciences attempted to resolve this disagreement by creating a commission to study DNA typing and determine its validity and reliability in forensic science. That commission issued its report, *DNA Technology in Forensic Science*, two years later. The report reviewed the status of DNA typing technology and its applications in forensic science and other fields. It gave special attention to both economic and ethical considerations involved in the use of DNA typing in forensic settings. While supporting the use of DNA typing in general and acknowledging that it was a potentially powerful tool of individualization, the committee hedged its conclusions and recommendations by warning of possible misuses of the technology. Its second recommendation, for example, was that

> *Prosecutors and defense counsel should not oversell DNA evidence. Presentations that suggest to a judge or jury that DNA typing is infallible are rarely justified and should be avoided.*[37]

In an effort to be evenhanded, the NRC commission may have failed to make its support of DNA typing strong enough and clear enough to end the debate among either experts or the general public. Defense lawyers, in fact, sometimes felt confident enough to continue challenging DNA evidence even to the extent of using the NRC report in support of their positions.

In the meanwhile, most of the scientific and law enforcement communities continued to have confidence in DNA typing and to develop and refine the technology on which the procedure is based and its application in court cases. In 1994, an article by Eric S. Lander and Bruce Budowle appeared in the journal *Nature* that appeared to resolve once and for all—at least for scientists—the status of DNA typing. "The DNA fingerprinting wars are over," the authors of that article wrote. ". . . the public needs to understand that the DNA fingerprinting controversy has been resolved. There is no scientific reason to doubt the accuracy of forensic DNA typing results, provided that the testing laboratory and the specific tests are on a par with currently practiced standards in the field. The scientific debates served a salutary purpose: standards were professionalized and research stimulated. But now it is time to move on."[38]

The key remaining issue—as it had always been—was human error. DNA tests are often carried out on very small samples of blood, hair, semen, or other materials. Even the smallest mistake can totally invalidate a test. As Eric S. Lander, then professor of biology at the Massachusetts Institute of Technology and director of the MIT Center for Genome Research said in a 1992 talk on DNA typing, " . . . if I sneeze on something, my DNA is there, too. And so there is tremendous need to avoid contamination."[39] This fact, Lander pointed out, requires that high standards of operation be established for DNA testing laboratories, and special efforts must be made to ensure that those laboratories abide by those standards.

DNA Databases

By the time the *Nature* article had appeared in 1994, confirming the scientific community's acceptance of DNA typing, law enforcement agencies had already accepted the validity of the technology and moved to incorporate it into their forensic toolboxes. One of the most powerful systems for using DNA profiles was the DNA database. A DNA database is simply a library of DNA samples taken from individuals and crime scenes and stored in some central location. The database is used to compare DNA samples collected at the scene of a crime or taken from people arrested for crimes with samples from known felons. It is also used to help solve so-called cold cases, which law enforcement officials have been unable to solve by any other means.

The FBI established the first DNA database in the United States in 1990 as a pilot project serving 14 state and local law enforcement laboratories. The success of that program led to the passage of the DNA Identification Act of 1994 (Public Law 103-322) that mandated the creation of a Combined DNA Index System (CODIS), a collaborative effort involving the FBI and state and local law enforcement agencies. The system is a three-tier program that makes possible the flow of information back and forth from local agencies (local DNA index systems; LDIS) to state agencies (state DNA index systems; SDIS) to the FBI (the National DNA Index System; NDIS), and back again.

The development of CODIS took place slowly, at least partly because all 50 states had to pass their own enabling legislation. The system became completely operational on November 14, 1998, although by that time CODIS had already been used to solve a number of crimes in participating states. (The first DNA database anywhere in the world was established in the United Kingdom on April 10, 1995.) As of 2007, CODIS contained DNA samples taken from more than 4 million convicted offenders and more than 160,000 crime scenes. The system had produced nearly 42,000 matches associated with about 43,000 criminal investigations in 49 states and two federal laboratories.

The success of CODIS tends to mask some ongoing issues about DNA databases. There is usually little dispute about the collection and storage of DNA samples from individuals convicted of violent crimes or from crime scenes. The problem is that some law enforcement officials and politicians have called for the expansion of DNA databases to include individuals who are arrested or accused of crimes, even if they are not prosecuted or convicted of those crimes. Former British prime minister Tony Blair was an especially enthusiastic proponent of expanding DNA databases to include anyone remotely involved in crime. In 2000, for example, he recommended increasing the U.K. DNA database to include "virtually the entire criminal population." That category would have included "anyone who is arrested on suspicion of any 'recordable' offense (including being drunk in a public place, begging, or taking part in a prohibited public procession), even though DNA evidence is usually not relevant to the investigation."[40] Similar proposals have come from a number of high-ranking officials in the

United States. In 2003, President George W. Bush proposed expanding the U.S. DNA database to include juvenile offenders and individuals who have been arrested for, but not necessarily tried for or convicted of, a crime. The likelihood was that the DNA database was likely to increase even further in the future. According to one official, Deborah Daniels, then assistant U.S. attorney general for justice programs: "DNA is to the 21st century what fingerprinting was to the 20th. The widespread use of DNA evidence is the future of law enforcement in this country."[41]

The argument in support of expanding DNA databases is that there is no way of knowing in advance who is going to commit a violent crime. If everyone's DNA is on file, solving an unexpected crime is likely to be much easier since critical evidence is already available in some DNA database. In addition, many proponents of expanding databases offer a familiar argument, namely that individuals who are not criminals should have no concern about providing DNA samples for law enforcement agencies.

On the other hand, suggestions for DNA databases that go beyond convicted criminals raise concern among civil libertarians. In the first place, a number of individuals accused of, suspected of, or arrested for crimes are never convicted of those crimes. They may be completely innocent persons who become enmeshed in the criminal justice system. Should their DNA become part of a database? And, if so, should the DNA of all innocent people be collected?

Also, critics ask, is it really necessary or helpful to expand DNA databases to include those convicted of nonviolent crimes, such as burglary, fraud, petty theft, or vagrancy? If so, should everyone convicted of a misdemeanor or felony be included in a DNA database, or are only certain types of crimes serious enough to be considered; if so, which crimes?

In an effort to solve this dilemma, Attorney General Janet Reno appointed a commission in 1998 to study DNA databases. That commission, the National Commission on the Future of DNA Evidence, consisted of scientists, law enforcement officials, prosecuting and defense attorneys, and judges. In its final report, the commission reviewed the scientific, political, legal, and ethical issues posed by DNA databases and identified yet another problem surrounding the expansion of such programs. Thus far, the commission discovered, DNA laboratories had been unable to keep up with the job of typing preexisting DNA samples of convicted felons. At the time the commission report was issued, nearly half a million DNA samples were still waiting to be typed and an equal number of convicted felons were waiting to have their DNA taken. Under these circumstances, the commission wrote, any proposals for the expansion of DNA databases were, for all practical purposes, moot.

DNA TYPING AS A TOOL FOR EXONERATING THE INNOCENT

For the general public, DNA typing has probably long been associated with the apprehension and conviction of violent criminals. Cases like that of Colin Pitchfork in England and Tommy Lee Andrews in the United States received national attention and showed the ordinary citizen what a powerful forensic tool DNA typing can be. But from its earliest days, DNA typing has also served a second function of equal importance: the determination of a person's innocence. In the Pitchfork case, for example, Alec Jeffreys was able to show that a confessed felon, Richard Buckland, was actually not guilty of the crime to which he had confessed.

In the United States, the first case in which DNA typing was used to establish a person's innocence involved Gary Dotson. Dotson had been convicted of rape in May 1979 and sentenced to 25 to 50 years in prison for the rape and an additional 25 to 50 years for aggravated assault. The decision and sentence were upheld by an appellant court in 1981. Six years later, the victim of the alleged crime confessed to her minister that she had lied about the rape because she feared that she had become pregnant by her boyfriend at the time. A lawyer hired on Dotson's behalf petitioned for his release and Illinois governor James R. Thompson commuted his sentence to time served, but did not revoke the original sentence. With the guilty verdict still on his record, Dotson remained on parole and was returned to prison in August 1987 when he was arrested on a charge of domestic violence against his live-in girlfriend. He remained in prison until August 14, 1989, when he was exonerated of the rape and aggravated assault charges on the basis of DNA evidence that proved his innocence. That evidence had become available exactly one year earlier, but it had taken the legal system a full 12 months to act on the new information and release Dotson from prison.

The Dotson case is only one example of dozens or hundreds of such cases that occur every year. All law enforcement officials know that wrongful convictions, terrible as they may be, are simply an inescapable part of the criminal justice system. People lie; they are confused; they seek revenge; they are mistaken about a person's identity; or they provide false information for some other reason, intentionally or not. No one knows how many falsely convicted men and women sit in America's prisons today. And until DNA typing was invented, there was virtually no way for such prisoners to prove their innocence.

Today, all that has changed. As the Gary Dotson case showed, DNA typing can provide absolute and incontrovertible evidence as to a person's innocence as well as it can prove one's guilt. In 1992, Barry Scheck and Peter Neufeld, defense attorneys in the case of *People v. Castro* founded the

Innocence Project to assist falsely convicted prisoners in proving their innocence by using DNA typing. The project is operated out of the Benjamin N. Cardozo School of Law at Yeshiva University in New York City. Most of the actual casework is conducted by students at the law school pro bono (at no charge) under the supervision of regular faculty members. Cases are selected from letters of application written by prisoners who believe they have a legitimate case for review.

As of 2007, the Innocence Project had been responsible for the release of more than 200 wrongfully convicted individuals. The longest-serving of these individuals is Paul Terry, who was convicted in 1977 of murder, aggravated kidnapping, rape, deviate sexual assault, and indecent liberties with a child, for which he was given a sentence of 400 years in prison. He was exonerated on the basis of DNA evidence in 2003 after serving 23 years of that sentence.

The success of the Innocence Project has led to the creation of similar organizations in 47 of the 50 states (the exceptions being Hawaii, North Dakota, and South Dakota), each of which works to discover evidence for individuals wrongfully convicted to crimes. In addition, many prisoners work on their own, with family and/or friends, or with other concerned individuals and organizations, to use DNA typing to overturn their convictions.

The Status of DNA Typing Today

The acceptance of DNA typing as a valid forensic technology with enormous power of discrimination occurred with astonishing speed. Scarcely 10 years after Alec Jeffreys invented the restriction fragment length polymorphism (RFLP) technique, DNA typing had become a routine and indispensable tool of law enforcement. By contrast, anthropometry has long since been abandoned as a method of individualization, ballistic fingerprinting and polygraph testing have received only limited acceptance, and questions are still being raised about the scientific validity of digital fingerprinting.

Since the mid-1990s, federal and state governments have focused on developing the legal infrastructure on which DNA typing is to be utilized in criminal cases. All 50 states now have sets of laws—diverse and inconsistent as they may be—dealing with individuals who are required to submit DNA samples, penalties for misuse of DNA information obtained in testing, specification of individuals and agencies who are authorized to see and use DNA data, and provisions for the retention of DNA samples and information obtained from those samples.

The keystone of federal DNA legislation is the Violent Crime Control and Law Enforcement Act of 1994 (VCCLEA), originally proposed as a set of amendments to the Omnibus Crime Control and Safe Streets Act of 1968. VCCLEA is best known for a number of topics unrelated to DNA typing, such as the ban on a number of types of weapons and funding for an increase in the number of police officers on the streets of the United States. Subtitle C of Section XXI of the act, however, provides the first comprehensive legislation on DNA typing in the United States. This section provides for funding of DNA laboratories in the United States, calls for the creation of standards for DNA typing in those laboratories, permits the creation of a DNA database by the Federal Bureau of Investigation (FBI), and establishes standards for the use of DNA typing by the FBI. VCCLEA provides the enabling legislation, therefore, for the FBI's Combined DNA Index System (CODIS).

The most recent major piece of federal legislation dealing with DNA testing was the 2004 Justice for All Act (Public Law 108-405). The purpose of the act was

> *[t]o protect crime victims' rights, to eliminate the substantial backlog of DNA samples collected from crime scenes and convicted offenders, to improve and expand the DNA testing capacity of Federal, State, and local crime laboratories, to increase research and development of new DNA testing technologies, to develop new training programs regarding the collection and use of DNA evidence, to provide postconviction testing of DNA evidence to exonerate the innocent, to improve the performance of counsel in State capital cases, and for other purposes.*[42]

The first part of the act, the Scott Campbell, Stephanie Roper, Wendy Preston, Louarna Gillis, and Nila Lynn Crime Victims' Rights Act, dealt with the rights of the victims of crime in general. The second part of the act, the Debbie Smith Act of 2004, focused on methods for reducing the backlog in cases of DNA typing awaiting completion and expansion of the FBI's CODIS database. The third part of the act, DNA Sexual Assault Justice Act of 2004, dealt with a number of miscellaneous issues related to DNA typing, including ensuring the compliance by public crime laboratory with federal standards; training and education in DNA typing for law enforcement, correctional personnel, and court officers; research and development on DNA typing; the use of DNA typing for identifying missing persons; and the establishment of penalties for improper use of DNA information. The fourth part of the act, the Innocence Protection Act of 2004, made a number of provisions for the use of DNA typing in the exoneration of prisoners wrongfully convicted of crimes, including grants to states to improve the quality of representation for such individuals and compensation to those who have been wrongfully incarcerated.

The discovery of DNA typing has marked a watershed in the history of forensic science. For centuries, those responsible for administering the law have searched for valid methods of proving that one specific individual, and no one else, was responsible for the commission of a crime. They have tried a host of procedures, ranging from trials of all sorts to the examination of bodily traits to fingerprinting, in that search. The discovery of RFLP by Alec Jeffreys in 1985 finally solved that problem. Today, no informed person any longer questions the validity and reliability of DNA typing as a virtually infallible method of forensic individualization. The law's long pursuit of a gold standard for identifying criminals has come to an end.

---

[1] Alphonse Bertillon, *Signaletic Instructions including the Theory and Practice of Anthropometrical Identification.* Chicago: The Werner Company, 1896, pp. 118–120.

[2] Bertillon, *Signaletic Instructions*, p. 61.

[3] As quoted in Simon A. Cole, *Suspect Identities: A History of Fingerprinting and Criminal Investigation.* Cambridge, Mass.: Harvard University Press, p. 58.

[4] Henry Faulds, "On the Skin-Furrows of the Hand," *Nature*, October 28, 1880, as reprinted by the Southern California Association of Fingerprint Officers. Available online. URL: http://www.scafo.org/library/100101.html. Accessed on May 10, 2007.

[5] Paul Rabinow, "Galton's Regret and DNA Typing," *Culture, Medicine, and Psychiatry*, vol. 17, no. 1, March 1993, pp. 59–65.

[6] Charles Féré, "Les Empreintes des Doigts et des Orteils," *Journal de l'Anatomie et de la Physiologie Normales et Pathologiques de l'Homme et des Animaux*, vol. 29, 1893, pp. 232–234, as cited in Simon A. Cole, "Fingerprint Identification and the Criminal Justice System: Historical Lessons for the DNA Debate," chapter 4 in David Lazer, ed. *DNA and the Criminal Justice System: The Technology of Justice.* Cambridge, Mass.: MIT Press, 2004.

[7] See note 3.

[8] Paul Gabriel Tesla, *Crime and Mental Disease in the Hand: A Proven Guide for the Identification and Pre-identification of Criminality, Psychosis and Mental Defectiveness.* Lakeland, Fla.: Osiris Press, 1991.

[9] David R. Ashbaugh, *Quantitative-Qualitative Friction Ridge Analysis: An Introduction to Basic and Advanced Ridgeology.* Boca Raton, Fla.: CRC Press, 1999, p. 138.

[10] Summarized in "'Daubert' Hearings." Available online. URL: http://www.ridgesandfurrows.homestead.com/radio_debate.html. Accessed on May 10, 2007.

[11] "Forensic Science Timeline," in Forensic Science. Available online. URL: http://www.umbc.edu/tele/canton/STUDENTPROJ/May.A/timeline.htm. Accessed on January 10, 2007.

[12] NIBIN Branch, Firearms Programs Division, Bureau of Alcohol, Tobacco, Firearms and Explosives. "ATF's NIBIN Program." Available online. URL: http://www.nibin.gov/nibin.pdf. Posted in December 2005.

[13] Lorraine Woellert, "Ballistics Fingerprinting: A Lifesaver." Business Week Online. Available online. URL: http://www.businessweek.com/bwdaily/dnflash/oct2002/nf20021024_3210.htm. Posted on October 24, 2002.

[14] Paul Magnusson, "Ballistics Fingerprinting: A Waste of Time." Business Week Online. Available online. URL: http://www.businessweek.com/bwdaily/dnflash/oct2002/nf20021024_9610.htm. Posted on October 24, 2002.

[15] John J. Tobin, Jr., "MD-IBIS Progress Report #2: Integrated Ballistics Identification System." Available online. URL: http://doubletap.cs.umd.edu/~purtilo/ibis.pdf. Posted in September 2004.

[16] Frederic A. Tulleners, "Technical Evaluation: Feasibility of a Ballistics Imaging Database for All New Handgun Sales." Sacramento and Santa Rosa Criminalistics Laboratories, Bureau of Forensic Services, California Department of Justice. Available online. URL: http://www.nssf.org/PDF/CA_study.pdf. Posted on October 5, 2001.

[17] Brady Campaign to Prevent Gun Violence, "Ballistic Fingerprints Help Solve Crimes." Available online. URL: http://www.bradycampaign.org/facts/issues/?page=ballistic. Accessed on July 2, 2007.

[18] Robert M. Thompson, Jerry Miller, Martin G. Ols, and Jennifer C. Budden, "Ballistic Imaging and Comparison of Crime Gun Evidence by the Bureau of Alcohol, Tobacco and Firearms." Washington, D.C.: Bureau of Alcohol, Tobacco, and Firearms, Department of the Treasury, May 13, 2002, p. 6.

[19] David B. Kopel and H. Sterling Burnett, "Ballistic Imaging: Not Ready for Prime Time." National Center for Policy Analysis. Policy Backgrounder No. 160. Available online. URL: http://www.ncpa.org/pub/bg/bg160/. Posted on April 30, 2003.

[20] Tulleners, p. 1.

[21] Quoted in Paul V. Trovillo, "A History of Lie Detection," *American Journal of Police Science*, vol. 29, no. 6, March–April 1939, p. 849.

[22] Quoted in Trovillo, p. 859.

[23] Quoted in Trovillo, p. 861.

[24] *Frye v. United States*, 54 App. D. C. 46, 293 F. 1013. The decision in this case can be found online. URL: http://www.daubertontheweb.com/frye_opinion.htm. Accessed on May 10, 2007.

[25] *Daubert v. Merrell Dow Pharmaceuticals*, 509 U.S. 579 (1993). The decision in this case can be found online. URL: http://supct.law.cornell.edu/supct/html/92-102.ZO.html. Accessed on May 10, 2007.

[26] *United States v. Scheffer*, 523 U.S. 303 (1998). The decision in this case can be found online. URL: http://supct.law.cornell.edu/supct/html/96-1133.ZS.html. Accessed on May 10, 2007.

[27] "Scientific Validity of Polygraph Testing: A Research Review and Evaluation—A Technical Memorandum." Washington, D. C.: U.S. Congress, Office of Technology Assessment, November 1983, p. 6.

[28] Committee to Review the Scientific Evidence on the Polygraph, Board on Behavioral, Cognitive, and Sensory Sciences and Committee on National Statistics, Division of Behavioral and Social Sciences and Education, National Research Council. *The Polygraph and Lie Detection*. Washington, D.C.: The National Academies Press, 2003, p. 2.

[29] Committee to Review the Scientific Evidence on the Polygraph, p. 4.

[30] "APA Response to the National Academy of Sciences (NAS) Report." Available online. URL: http://www.polygraph.org/nasresponse.htm. Accessed on February 28, 2007.

[31] The law can be found in Massachusetts General Laws, Chapter 149, Section 19B. Available online. URL: http://www.mass.gov/legis/laws/mgl/149-19b.htm. Accessed on May 10, 2007.

[32] "Semiannual Report to Congress." Available online. URL: http://www.usdoj.gov/oig/semiannual/0611/index.htm. Accessed on February 28, 2007.

[33] Nick Zagorski, "Profile of Alec J. Jeffreys," *Proceedings of the National Academy of Sciences*, vol. 103, no. 24, June 13, 2006, p. 8919.

[34] Ron Fridell, *DNA Fingerprinting: The Ultimate Identity*. New York: Franklin Watts, 2001, p. 36.

[35] *United States v. Jakobetz*, 955 F.2d 786 (2nd Cir. 01/09/1992). Available online. URL: http://www.cjcentral.com/jakobetz.htm. Accessed on February 28, 2007.

[36] Howard Coleman and Eric Swenson, *DNA in the Courtroom: A Trial Watcher's Guide*. Seattle, Wash.: GenLex Press, 1994, p. 5; as quoted in Fridell, p. 35.

[37] Committee on DNA Technology in Forensic Science, Board on Biology, Commission on Life Sciences, National Research Council, *DNA Technology in Forensic Science*. Washington, D.C.: National Academy Press, p. 161.

[38] Eric S. Lander and Bruce Budowle, "DNA Fingerprinting, Dispute Laid to Rest," *Nature*, vol. 371, no. 6500, October 27, 1994, pp. 735, 738.

[39] "Use of DNA in Identification." Access Excellence @ the National Health Museum. Available online. URL: http://www.accessexcellence.org/RC/AB/BA/Use_of_DNA_Identification.html. Accessed on February 28, 2007.

[40] Tania Simoncelli and Helen Wallace, "Expanding Databases, Declining Liberties." Council for Responsible Genetics. Available online. URL: http://www.gene-watch.org/genewatch/articles/19-1TSHW.html. Accessed on February 28, 2007.

[41] Richard Willing, "White House Seeks to Expand DNA Database." *USA Today*. Available online. URL: http://www.usatoday.com/news/washington/2003-04-15-dna-usat_x.htm. Posted on April 15, 2003.

[42] H.R. 1507. Available online. URL: http://thomas.loc.gov/cgi-bin/bdquery/z?d108:h.r.05107:. Accessed on March 5, 2007.

CHAPTER 2

THE LAW RELATING TO FORENSIC SCIENCE AND DNA EVIDENCE

The chapter describes laws, legislative actions, administration rulings, and legal decisions relating to anthropometry, fingerprinting, ballistic analysis, polygraph testing, and DNA typing conducted in the United States. Extracts from some of these laws, court decisions, and other legal documents appear in the Appendices.

FEDERAL LAWS AND ADMINISTRATIVE ACTIONS

FEDERAL RULES OF EVIDENCE (1975)

A fundamental part of every legal case is evidence, that collection of documents, material objects, written and oral records, and testimony presented by both sides in a case. One of the basic decisions that must be made in every court case is which pieces of evidence are admissible and which are not. That is, the presiding judge must always decide whether he or she or the jury will be allowed to hear or see any given piece of evidence.

Prior to 1975, no single federal standard was available to determine the admissibility of evidence. Courts relied on case law, decisions that had been made in previous cases relevant to the one being considered, or common law, legal "truths" that had been handed down throughout legal history. During the 20th century, however, the federal government and a number of individual states had begun to develop standards for the admissibility of evidence. Some of the most important of these efforts were the Uniform Rules of Evidence, adopted in 1974; the Federal Rules of Civil Procedure, first promulgated in 1938 by the U.S. Supreme Court; and the California

Evidence Code, first adopted in 1965. (The Uniform Rules of Evidence is a set of standards established by the National Conference of Commissioners on Uniform State Laws, a group of lawyers who offer advice to the individual states on the drafting of laws.)

In 1965, Chief Justice Earl Warren appointed a committee of 15 legal experts to draw up a new set of federal standards for the admissibility of evidence. The committee presented drafts in 1969, 1971, and 1972 for public comment, but a final decision was not reached until three years later when Congress finally allowed the new Federal Rules of Evidence (FRE) to become law.

FRE consists of 67 separate rules arranged in 11 categories, such as relevancy and its limits, privileges, witnesses, opinions and expert testimony, and hearsay. One of the most important rules relating to forensic science is Rule 702, which says that:

> *If scientific, technical, or other specialized knowledge will assist the trier of fact to understand the evidence or to determine a fact in issue, a witness qualified as an expert by knowledge, skill, experience, training, or education, may testify thereto in the form of an opinion or otherwise, if (1) the testimony is based upon sufficient facts or data, (2) the testimony is the product of reliable principles and methods, and (3) the witness has applied the principles and methods reliably to the facts of the case.*[1]

This standard is somewhat more liberal than that set by *Frye v. United States* in 1923, then the determining standard for the admissibility of evidence. The *Frye* standard said that scientific evidence could be admitted in a case if a principle, technique, or procedure had been "generally accepted" within the relevant field. The results of polygraph testing, for example, the technology involved in the *Frye* case, could be accepted if the technology of polygraph testing had been widely accepted within the scientific community (which, the court decided in *Frye*, it had not). According to the FRE standard, evidence could be admitted if a witness was qualified to discuss a principle, procedure, or technology even if that principle, procedure, or technology had not yet been widely adopted within the scientific community. The impact of FRE on admissibility of evidence was to become most apparent two decades after the adoption of the new rules of evidence, in the pivotal Supreme Court decision of *Daubert v. Merrell Dow Pharmaceutical.*

Employee Polygraph Protection, United States Code (1988)

In 1988, the U.S. Congress passed the Employee Polygraph Protection Act, Public Law 100-347. That act became part of Title 29 of the United States

Code and established federal regulations about the use of polygraph testing by employers. It applies to "polygraph, deceptograph, voice stress analyzer, psychological stress evaluator, or any other similar device (whether mechanical or electrical)" that is used to determine the veracity of a subject's statements made in interviews with employees or prospective employees. The act prohibits the use of such instruments for the purpose of making hiring decisions, for investigating or releasing employees, or to discriminate against employees or prospective employees in any other way. Exemptions are granted to employees of the federal, state, and local governments; in situations where national security is an issue; and for use by certain specific governmental agencies, such as the Federal Bureau of Investigation (FBI). Employers who violate the provisions of this act are subject to legal action by injured individuals and to fines not to exceed $10,000.

MILITARY RULE OF EVIDENCE 707, POLYGRAPH TESTING (1991)

In 1975, the U.S. Congress approved the adoption of the Federal Rules of Evidence (FRE), a set of rules dealing with the admissibility of evidence presented in federal court cases. Five years later, President Jimmy Carter promulgated a similar document dealing with military law, known as the Military Rules of Evidence (MRE). MRE has been modified and expanded on a number of occasions since its adoption in 1980. One such change, dealing with polygraph testing, was authorized by President George H. W. Bush in 1991. That rule bars the admission of polygraph results, the opinion of the polygraph examiner, or any reference to an offer to take, failure to take, or taking of a polygraph examination in courts-martial. The rule was first tested in 1996 in the case of *United States v. Scheffer*, 41 M.J. 683. In that case, defendant Scheffer claimed the right to submit evidence collected during a polygraph test for which he volunteered. Both the military trial court and the Air Force Court of Criminal Appeals rejected Scheffer's claim, basing their decisions on the provision of Rule 707. The United States Court of Appeals for the Armed Forces overturned those decisions in 1997, however, declaring that Rule 707 is unconstitutional. The case finally advanced to the U.S. Supreme Court in 1998, which, in an 8 to 1 ruling, declared Rule 707 to be constitutional. The rule has continued to provide the guiding principle on polygraph testing in the military to the present day.

REGULATION AND CODIFICATION OF DNA TESTING (1994)

On September 13, 1994, President Bill Clinton signed an act of Congress amending the Omnibus Crime Control and Safe Streets Act of 1968. The act made a number of changes in the original act, including authorizing grants to increase the number of police officers hired by local departments, expanding and improving cooperative efforts between law enforcement agencies and members of the community to address crime and disorder problems, and regulating and codifying the testing of DNA samples in the nation's forensic laboratories. The act became Public Law 103-322 and is codified in the United States Code, Title 42, chapter 136, sections 14131 through 14133.

The first of the three sections requires the Federal Bureau of Investigation (FBI) to establish standards for DNA laboratories to ensure that their work meets reasonable scientific criteria for such research. The section also calls for the hiring of an independent firm to do so-called blind external proficiency testing of DNA laboratories. Blind external proficiency testing is testing carried out by some authenticating agency to determine the proficiency of a testing laboratory's work without that laboratory's knowing the real purpose for which the test is being conducted. Finally, the section calls for the creation of an advisory board of scientific experts in the field of DNA typing to advise the FBI on technical questions relating to DNA testing.

The second section of the act provides for the creation of a DNA "index" that contains DNA records obtained by both federal and state agencies consisting of four kinds of records: (1) those collected from persons convicted of crimes; (2) those recovered from crime scenes; (3) those recovered from unidentified human remains; and (4) those voluntarily contributed from relatives of missing persons. The section also provides for a system by which federal and state governments can exchange DNA records with each other.

The third section of the act deals specifically with standards and procedures for DNA typing conducted by members of the FBI. It sets standards for the training of such individuals, provides for their blind external proficiency testing, and clarifies privacy requirements for individuals for whom DNA samples are collected. The section also prescribes penalties for government employees who violate any provision of this section of the act.

FEDERAL LEGISLATION ON BALLISTIC FINGERPRINTING (2002)

The proliferation of guns in American society is a matter of some concern to many people. Guns are involved in tens of thousands of violent crimes every year. Some people advocate the use of ballistic fingerprinting as a way of tracing weapons used in such crimes and identifying the people responsible for them. The principles of ballistic fingerprinting, these people say, are well known, and they can be used to track down the owners of weapons used in violent crimes. They recommend the establishment of a national database that contains ballistic markings for all weapons manufactured in the United States and, in some cases, imported into the country. Such a database would be similar to databases for digital and DNA fingerprints already operated by the federal and many state governments.

As of 2006, two states—New York and Maryland—have adopted laws establishing such databases. The Maryland law, for example, requires gun manufacturers to test-fire the handguns they make and to send to the state police a spent shell casing from each gun sold in the state. Similar legislation has been introduced at the federal level on a number of occasions. Perhaps the best known bills were Senate bill S. 3096, written by Senator Herb Kohl (D-Wis.), and House bill H.R. 5663, introduced by Representative Anita Eshoo (D-Calif.). Both bills contained identical wording and were introduced in 2002 in the 107th Congress. The bills would have required all gun manufacturers and importers to testfire the weapons they make and sell, prepare ballistic images of the bullets and cartridge casings, provide permanent storage for those bullets and cartridges, and transmit the records of these tests to the Bureau of Alcohol, Tobacco and Firearms (ATF). The bill also requires the ATF to establish a computerized database that federal, state, and local law enforcement agencies can access, and allocated $20 million to fund the program's operation.

The bills were introduced shortly after and partly in response to a series of sniper killings that took place in the Washington, D.C., area in 2002. Some experts argued that the availability of a ballistics database might have made apprehension of the snipers easier and saved a number of lives. Other experts disagreed. The biggest problem with the Kohl and Eshoo bills, they pointed out, was that more than 250 million guns were already in the hands of Americans, and it was inconceivable that owners would cooperate with a ballistics testing program that would allow registration of those guns in the national database. In any case, the Kohl and Eshoo bills failed and similar legislation has not been introduced. The Maryland and New York laws remain on the books although they too are subject to severe criticism. In 2005, for example, Colonel Thomas E. Hutchins, superintendent of the Maryland State Police, recommended that the state ballistic fingerprinting law be repealed. He pointed out that more than $2 million had already been spent on the program without achieving a single conviction.

PRESIDENT'S DNA INITIATIVE (2003)

By the beginning of the 21st century, DNA typing had become widely accepted by forensic scientists and law enforcement officials as one of the most valid and reliable methods of identifying an individual involved in a crime. One remaining problem with the use of DNA typing, however, was the delay involved in collecting, analyzing, and interpreting DNA samples collected from an individual or a crime scene. In August 2001, Attorney General John Ashcroft decided to attack this problem. He directed the National

Institute of Justice (NIJ) to develop recommendations for ways of reducing the delay involved in the use of DNA typing. In response to this charge, the NIJ convened a working group consisting of experts in forensic science and DNA typing from local, state, and national levels. That group submitted a report to the Attorney General in late 2002 that became the basis of the President's DNA Initiative and a group of bills dealing with the use of DNA technology in law enforcement.

President George W. Bush announced his President's DNA Initiative on March 11, 2003. The initiative calls for the investment of more than $1 billion for funding, training, and assistance of federal, state, and local forensic laboratories and law enforcement personnel with the goal of ensuring that DNA typing is used to its greatest potential in solving crimes, protecting the innocent, and identifying missing persons. The initiative was given the name Advancing Justice through DNA Technology. The initiative has a number of specific objectives, including elimination of the backlog of unanalyzed DNA samples, improvement of crime laboratories' efficiency in analyzing DNA samples, stimulation of research on new DNA technologies, development of training programs for technicians who work with DNA evidence, and access to DNA testing not present or made available at a trial.

The NIJ report was also instrumental in the adoption of legislation that dovetailed with the President's DNA Initiative. The most important of that legislation was H.R. 5107, the Justice for All Act, introduced on September 21, 2004, by Representative F. James Sensenbrenner, Jr. (R-Wis.). The bill was passed by the House of Representatives on October 6, by the Senate on October 9, and signed into law by President Bush on October 30, 2004, when it became Public Law 108405. The law provided directives and funding to the Department of Justice and other agencies with the goal of carrying out many of the objectives stated by President Bush in his March 2003 announcement of the President's DNA Initiative.

STATE LAWS (2007)

All 50 states and the federal government now require that individuals implicated or convicted of certain crimes submit DNA samples to law enforcement agencies. These samples are then tested, typed, and entered into state and national DNA databases. The results of these DNA typings are then retained in the databases in all cases essentially forever, with no provisions for deletion of the information upon the criminal's having completed his or her sentence or other punishment.

State laws have evolved over a period of almost two decades in a variety of directions, resulting in a crazy quilt array of DNA statutes throughout the 50 states and the federal government. In general, those laws fall into four general categories: (1) designation of those individuals who are required to submit DNA samples; (2) provision of penalties for misuse of DNA information obtained in such tests; (3) specification of those individuals and agencies who are authorized to see and use DNA data; and (4) provisions for the retention of DNA samples and information obtained from those samples. States may have laws in any one or more of these four categories. In many cases, they have more than one law dealing with any specific topic.

At one time, DNA typing was required by state laws only for individuals convicted of certain crimes. That practice spread rapidly, however, and as of 2007, 34 states had statutes requiring anyone convicted of a felony to submit a DNA sample. Many states (38 in 2007) also require DNA typing for certain types of misdemeanor crimes, usually those in which violence or sex is involved. More recently some states have required DNA typing for individuals who have been arrested of a crime, whether or not they have been tried and/or convicted of the crime or not. As of 2007, seven states—California, Kansas, Louisiana, Minnesota, New Mexico, Texas, and Virginia—along with the federal government have laws for the testing of DNA from arrestees as well as from those convicted of a crime. A number of other states are considering legislation to include arrestees in their DNA statutes, and this movement appears to be gaining momentum in the nation. Consideration for the arrestee who is judged innocent is reflected in the fact that most states with arrestee laws—Louisiana, New Mexico, Texas, and Virginia—require that DNA information be discarded if a person is found innocent of a crime.

Another recent trend in state statutes has been the adoption of laws allowing and describing the conditions for post-conviction DNA testing. Such laws permit a person who has been convicted of a crime, usually whether or not the conviction involved the use of DNA typing, to request a DNA analysis of evidence available in the case. The laws have been passed to some extent as a result of the advocacy of the Innocence Project, an organization that works to assist innocent individuals who have unfairly been convicted of crimes they did not commit. As of 2007, about two dozen states had post-conviction DNA laws that, like other DNA laws, differ from each other in some substantial ways. The major differences among these laws have to do with who it is that can apply for DNA testing; who pays for the tests; whether preservation of samples and results is required and, if so, under what conditions; and who pays for preservation of the samples and results. Given the fairly large number of individuals who have been freed as the result of DNA testing (about 200 as of 2007), it is reasonable to assume that post-conviction DNA testing laws are likely to become more popular in the future.

COURT CASES

PEOPLE V. JENNINGS, 252 ILL. 534, 96 N.E. 1077 (1911)

Background

On the evening of September 10, 1910, 15-year-old Clarice Hiller was awakened in her Church Street home in Chicago, Illinois, by an intruder who lifted her nightgown and touched her body. After the girl screamed for help, the intruder attempted to flee, however, he encountered the girl's father, Clarence Hiller. After a short struggle between the two men, the intruder shot Hiller in the neck, killing him instantly. Thirteen minutes later, Thomas Jennings was apprehended by four off-duty members of the Chicago Police Department when they noticed blood stains on Jennings's shirt. Investigators discovered a clear set of fingerprints on the recently painted porch railing at the Hiller home. When Jennings was fingerprinted by the police, his prints were found to match those found on the porch railing. At Jennings's subsequent trial for the murder of Hiller, five fingerprint experts testified that the two sets of prints matched. Based largely on this evidence, Jennings was convicted of Hiller's murder. The defense then appealed the decision, and the case eventually reached the Illinois Supreme Court.

Legal Issues

The *People v. Jennings* is a significant case in the history of fingerprinting, because it is the first occasion on which the validity and reliability of fingerprints as forensic evidence was decided by the highest court in a state. At the initial trial, the defense had argued that no experts were necessary to examine and identify Jennings's prints and those found at the scene of the crime. All that was needed, the defense argued, was for members of the jury to look at the prints through a microscope and draw their own conclusions about a possible match. The trial judge disagreed. He pointed out that fingerprint analysis had become a widely accepted scientific procedure in which some individuals had special expertise. He agreed with the prosecution's argument that a general consensus within the scientific community existed that fingerprints truly are unique and that differences among individuals' fingerprints provided a legitimate basis for making identifications.

Decision

When it reviewed the lower court's ruling on the Hiller murder, the Illinois Supreme Court essentially agreed with the trial judge's view on the admissibility of fingerprint evidence. It concluded that fingerprints had been used for the purpose of identification for a long time and that the scientific community was in general agreement that fingerprints were as unique as snowflakes. The court said in its opinion that "there is a scientific basis for the system of fingerprint identification and that the courts are justified in admitting this class of evidence."[2] At the same time, the court made it clear that the status of fingerprint evidence made it not only reasonable, but also essential that experts in the field be permitted to testify in cases in which such evidence was presented. The supreme court affirmed the lower court's decision and sentenced Jennings to death on February 16, 1912.

Impact

People v. Jennings is one of the classic cases in forensic science because it established a legal precedent that has lasted for almost a century. Virtually all legal cases in which fingerprint evidence is presented as evidence rest, either explicitly or implicitly, on the rulings made in *People v. Jennings*. Only in the last decade or so have defense attorneys once more begun to question the scientific validity of the argument that fingerprints of different individuals are sufficiently unique to allow them to be used for the identification of individuals in criminal cases. Thus far, these objections to the use of fingerprint evidence have received almost no favorable response by the courts.

STATE V. KUHL, 42 NEV. 185, 175 PACIFIC 190 (1918)

Background

On December 5, 1916, the stagecoach from Rogerson, Idaho, to Jarbidge, Nevada, was three hours late, prompting local officials to launch a search for the coach. About an hour later, the search party found the missing coach and its driver, whose throat had been slashed. The mail sacks had been cut open and $4,000 in gold Double Eagle coins were missing. A black overcoat was recovered at the crime scene and soon connected with Ben Kuhl, who had worked as a cook at the local OK mine. Kuhl already had a criminal record and was arrested on suspicion of having committed the robbery and murder. His trial was held on September 8, 1917.

Legal Issues

Most of the evidence against Ben Kuhl was circumstantial. A number of witnesses recalled that he was often seen wearing a black overcoat with tears in the sleeves similar to the one found at the scene of the crime. A positive identification of the coat's belonging to Kuhl was not made, however. Instead, the pivotal evidence turned out to be a bloody palm print found on an envelope found at the scene of the crime. Two fingerprint experts from California, Charles H. Stone and O. W. Bottoroff, testified that the palm print matched one taken from Kuhl while he was being held in jail. The prosecutor argued that this match was sufficient to prove that Kuhl had committed the robbery and the murder. The issue facing the court was that, while fingerprints had been admitted into evidence for many years in both the United States and other countries, palm prints had never been offered in evidence before. The court had to decide whether palm prints had the same unique properties as fingerprints.

Decision

On October 6, 1917, the jury found Ben Kuhl guilty of all charges lodged against him. It announced that the palm print evidence was critical in its decision. Kuhl was sentenced to death and given the choice of hanging or death by firing squad. He chose the latter and was sentenced to die on January 10, 1918. One week before the sentence was carried out, the governor of Nevada intervened, asking the Nevada Supreme Court to review the case. The court affirmed the lower court's decision and sentenced Kuhl to die on December 20, 1918. In announcing the court's decision justice Patrick A. McCarran noted that the Kuhl case was the first instance in which palm print, rather than fingerprint, evidence was presented as a means of identification. The court had decided, however, that "[a]ll of the learned authors, experts, and scientists on the subject of finger print identification, and each of those to whom we have heretofore referred, agree that these patterns, formed by the papillary ridges on the inner surface of the human hand and the sole of the foot, are persistent, continuous, and unchanging from a period in the existence of the individual extending from some months before birth until disintegration after death."[3] Palm prints could be considered, therefore, as reliable a form of personal identification as fingerprints. (As a point of interest, Kuhl's death sentence was commuted a week before he was scheduled to die, and he was given instead a life sentence. He was paroled in 1943 and died a year later.)

Impact

The significance of *State v. Kuhl* is simple and specific: It set the precedent that palm prints were as valid as fingerprints for purposes of identifying individuals in criminal cases. That principle was also extended to toe and foot prints in 1934 in the case of *People v. Les*, 267 Michigan 648, 255 NW 407.

FRYE V. UNITED STATES, 54 APP. D. C. 46, 293 F. 1013 (1923)

Background

Credit for the invention of the first modern polygraph is often given to John Larson, a police officer with the Berkeley, California, police department in about 1921. One of the first cases in which the polygraph was used involved the murder of Dr. Robert W. Brown, a black physician in Berkeley. Although the murderer was seen fleeing the scene of the crime by another physician in Brown's office, the witness was unable to identify the suspect. Seven months later, James Frye was arrested for an unrelated crime and, during the investigation of that crime, he also confessed to the murder of Dr. Brown. The precise details relating to Frye's confession have long been the subject of some dispute. In any case, he later withdrew his confession and said that he had not been involved in the Brown murder. During the ongoing investigation of the crime, Frye was asked to take a polygraph test about his confession, the results of which indicated that Frye's statement of innocence was, in fact, true and that he had not murdered Dr. Brown. When Frye was tried for the murder, his attorney attempted to introduce evidence from the polygraph test in his defense.

Legal Issues

The primary issue facing the trial court was whether the polygraph test taken by Frye was admissible in the Brown murder case. At the time, no previous legal challenges to polygraph testing had arisen. Indeed, polygraph evidence had never been offered in a criminal case before. The trial court was faced with the challenge, then, of making a de novo decision as to the legality of polygraph testing.

Decision

Given its historic significance, the court's decision in *Frye v. United States* is remarkably brief and lacking in annotations. The court pointed out that the fundamental issue to be decided was the point at which some new technology "crosses the line between the experimental and demonstrable stages." It also noted that courts have a difficult time in determining when that point has been reached, and they must rely on the testimony of experts in the field as to when a technology has gained general acceptance. At that point, evidence produced by the technology can be accepted by the courts.

Impact

Frye is one of the most important cases in forensic science because it set a standard for the admissibility of evidence that remained in effect for seven decades. After the *Frye* ruling, courts adopted the standard of "general acceptance" within the relevant field in determining whether or not evidence could be admitted. That standard meant that an attorney would have to show that some procedure, technique, or principle had been widely accepted and adopted within a field in order for courts to accept evidence on which it was based. In the case of polygraph testing, the "general acceptance" test meant that anyone wishing to offer polygraph data in evidence would first have to show that polygraph testing was widely accepted within the field of forensic science as providing reliable and valid information as to whether a person is telling the truth or not. As of the early 21st century, polygraph testing has still not attained that status, and evidence obtained from testing is still almost universally excluded from legal testimony.

People v. George Wesley, 533 N.Y.S.2d 643 (1988)

Background

On September 15, 1987, a 79-year-old woman, Helen Kendrick, was found dead in her apartment in the city of Albany, New York. George Wesley was implicated in the crime when caseworkers from the Albany City Hostel made a routine check of his apartment. Both Kendrick and Wesley were clients served by the hostel, an organization that serves developmentally disabled individuals. Caseworkers found a bloodstained T-shirt with gray and white hairs on it, bloodstained underwear, and bloodstained sweatpants. Investigators for the local police department rather easily developed a strong case against Wesley, and he was charged with the murder of Kendrick. As part of their investigations, the police tested the suspect's clothing for a DNA profile and found that it matched one taken from Wesley. Wesley was tried in the county court for Albany and found guilty. He appealed the decision based partly on his belief that the DNA results used in his conviction were unreliable, DNA typing being a new and relatively untested forensic technology.

Legal Issues

Wesley's appeal was heard by the New York Court of Appeals in 1994. The court commented that the DNA results produced by the prosecution were a relatively unimportant factor in the trial court's decision, writing that "[e]ven without the DNA profiling evidence, proof of defendant's guilt is compelling." Nonetheless, it heard extensive testimony on the technology of DNA typing and released an extended opinion dealing with the admissibility of evidence obtained from the procedure. The primary issue faced by the court was whether DNA typing had advanced to a point where it was generally accepted by the scientific community as a valid and reliable method of connecting an individual with a specific DNA sample, as provided for by the so-called *Frye* standard of evidence then in force in the legal community.

Decision

After consideration of the scientific evidence about DNA typing and reviewing the records of the trial court procedure, the appeals court decided that DNA fingerprinting met the standards for admissibility established by *Frye*. The court wrote that "[w]e hold that since DNA evidence was found to be generally accepted as reliable by the relevant scientific community and since a proper foundation was made at trial, DNA profiling evidence was properly admitted at trial." The appeals court denied Wesley's appeal and his sentence of life imprisonment was confirmed.

Impact

Wesley is of major significance in the history of DNA typing in the United States because it was the first upper-level court decision in which the scientific validity of DNA typing was confirmed. Since that decision, almost all courts in which DNA evidence has been presented have cited *Wesley* or implicitly accepted its arguments as providing the necessary basis for its admissibility in a criminal case. The fundamental standard for admissibility, *Frye*, has since been replaced by a newer standard, the *Daubert* standard (see below). The existence of this new standard has had no effect, however, on the unanimous view of courts that DNA typing is a valid and reliable scientific technique that produces results that are admissible in a court case.

State of Florida v. Tommy Lee Andrews, 533 So. 2d 841 (Fla. Dist Ct. App.) (1988)

Background

On February 22, 1986, a man broke into the home of Nancy Hodges in Orlando, Florida, and repeatedly raped and assaulted her. The assailant covered his victim with a sleeping bag to prevent her from identifying him, but he left two fingerprints on the window screen as he left the Hodges' home. Over the next year, 23 more cases of a similar nature were reported in the Orlando area. Finally, on March 1, 1987, Orlando police apprehended Tommy Lee Andrews, a 24-year-old warehouse worker, and charged him with two counts of rape, one being that of Nancy Hodges. Andrews was brought to trial for the Hodges rape on October 27, 1987. In a pre-trial hearing, the prosecution had proposed offering evidence from DNA typing on samples collected at the crime scene and from Andrews.

Legal Issues

The prosecution decided to introduce DNA evidence in the Andrews trial having heard of the recent use of the technology in the murder conviction of Colin Pitchfork in Leicester, England, in January 1987. At that point, DNA typing had never been presented in a U.S. court and the prosecution's first task was to convince the judge that the technology was sufficiently advanced to allow its use in a trial. The judge agreed to allow the DNA evidence to be used.

Decision

When the prosecutor presented the DNA evidence linking Andrews to the Hodges rape during the trial, he made a serious miscalculation. He said that the chances of an incorrect match was only one in 10 billion. When asked to provide scientific evidence for that figure, he was unable to do so and had to withdraw the evidence. Unconvinced by the DNA evidence or any other testimony provided at the trial, the jury was unable to reach a decision and the judge declared a mistrial.

Two weeks later, a second trial was held in which Andrews was accused of raping a second woman under circumstances similar to those in the Hodges case. The prosecutor once more offered DNA testing results in evidence, but this time provided statistical reasons for trusting in the test results. This time the jury was convinced, and they found Andrews guilty of rape and sentenced him to 22 years in prison. In a February 1988 retrial of the Hodges rape, DNA evidence was submitted once more, again with sound scientific support by the prosecution. Again the jury was convinced by the evidence and Andrews was sentenced to an additional 78 years for rape, 22 years for burglary, and 15 years for battery. Upon appeal, the Florida District Court of Appeals upheld the lower court's findings, including its decision to allow DNA results as evidence in the case.

Impact

Tommy Lee Andrews was the first person in the United States to be convicted based primarily on DNA evidence. Acceptance of the admissibility of DNA evidence by the trial and appellate courts set a precedent that many other courts later used to justify admission of DNA typing in court cases.

People v. Castro, 545 NYS 2d 985 (1989)

Background

On February 5, 1987, Bronx resident Vilma Ponce and her two-year-old daughter, Natasha, were stabbed to death in their apartment. The primary suspect in the case was Jose Castro, a neighbor of Ponce. Castro had been seen leaving the apartment building, covered in blood, by Ponce's partner, David Rivera, as he returned home from work. When Castro returned to his apartment two days later, Rivera called the police and identified Castro as the possible murderer of his partner and young child. Circumstantial evidence pointed to Castro as the possible perpetrator of the crime, but it was not strong enough to make a convincing case against him. The prosecution decided to rely heavily on a small sample of blood found on Castro's watch that they claimed came from Ponce. DNA tests were conducted on the blood and on a sample of tissue taken from Castro. The samples appeared to match.

Legal Issues

By the time of the Castro trial, DNA typing had become a widely accepted forensic technique in the United States and other parts of the world. It had then been used as evidence in 80 murder and rape cases in 27 states and had never been seriously challenged by defense attorneys. Nonetheless, expert witnesses were called by both prosecution and defense to support or refute the validity of DNA test results in this particular case. As the trial progressed, it became clear to both sides that the DNA tests prepared for the court were of dubious quality. In a somewhat unprecedented move, the judge asked four expert witnesses from both sides to meet and jointly analyze the DNA data available to them. The four experts eventually came to the conclusion that the quality of the DNA samples was insufficient to permit any conclusions. They so reported to the judge, and he excluded the DNA tests from the trial.

Decision

Lacking the DNA evidence that she thought would conclusively resolve the case for her, the prosecutor instead offered Castro a plea bargain, offering him a sentence of 20 years to life rather than taking a chance on the death sentence that would result from a conviction. Castro accepted the bargain, and later confessed to the murder of Ponce and her child.

Impact

As would be obvious, the decision in *People v. Castro* emboldened other defense attorneys in other venues to raise questions about the validity and reliability of DNA testing. In the long run, most of the objections to DNA testing failed, largely because of the major consequence of the case. The problem in *People v. Castro* was not DNA testing itself, but the care with which it was done. The company responsible for preparing DNA samples for the Castro case had simply been too careless, producing results that could not be read with sufficient clarity to allow a definite conclusion to be drawn. That company later improved its own technology, as did other companies involved in DNA testing, so that there is essentially no longer any dispute about the legitimacy of DNA typing in the identification of individuals.

UNITED STATES V. JAKOBETZ, 955 F.2D 786 (1992)

Background

On June 13, 1989, a young woman traveling on Interstate 91 in Vermont stopped at a rest area to use the restroom. As she was leaving the restroom, a man attacked her, tied her up, and placed her in the back of a semi-trailer truck. He drove down the highway for some distance before stopping at another rest stop, getting into the back of the truck, and raping the woman repeatedly and brutally. He then returned to the cab of the truck and drove farther south on the highway. He eventually released the woman at yet another rest stop farther south. Based on evidence provided by the victim and telephone records of calls made at the first rest stop, police were able to identify Randolph Jakobetz as a suspect in the crime. When police searched Jakobetz's truck, they found physical evidence linking him with the victim. Eventually, DNA obtained from a blood test on Jakobetz was also found to match DNA taken from semen on the woman's clothing. He was tried in the U.S. District Court for Vermont and found guilty on October 1, 1990. Jakobetz appealed the verdict based on a number of procedural rulings made by the trial judge, the most important of which was his decision to allow the use of DNA evidence by the prosecution.

Legal Issues

The appeals court reviewed the history of DNA typing in forensic cases and chose to focus on the decision in *People v. Castro* as an important precedent in its own deliberations. It pointed out that the judge in *Castro* established a three-prong criterion for the admissibility of scientific evidence: (1) the existence of a theory that is generally accepted in the scientific community and that supports the conclusion that DNA typing can produce reliable results; (2) the existence of techniques or experiments that are capable of producing reliable results and that are generally accepted by the scientific community; and (3) confirmation that the testing laboratory that has prepared the DNA evidence has followed accepted scientific techniques in analyzing the forensic samples. The court in this case pointed out that the first two points are embedded in both the traditional standard for the admissibility of scientific evidence (*Frye*, above) and the Federal Rules of Evidence (FRE), which had largely superceded *Frye* at the time of this trial. It concluded, then, that the remaining issue was whether the testing laboratory had met the third prong of the *Castro* test before the DNA evidence was presented by the prosecution.

Decision

The appeals court concluded that the district court judge had acted properly in assuring that the DNA evidence presented in the Jakobetz case was properly obtained. It wrote that "[w]e thus conclude that the district court properly exercised its discretion in admitting the DNA profiling evidence proffered by the government in this case." Significantly, the court went on to establish a general principle for the use of DNA typing evidence. It concluded that such evidence was now well confirmed by the scientific community and there was no longer any question as to its validity or its admissibility in criminal trials. In its decision, the court wrote that "we also conclude that courts facing a similar issue in the future can take judicial notice of the general theories and specific techniques involved in DNA profiling."[4] The U.S. Supreme Court declined to hear an appeal of the appeals court ruling, so its decision now stands as an important standard in the admissibility of DNA evidence.

Impact

Jakobetz is of major significance in the legal history of DNA typing because it clearly confirmed the validity of the technique as a reliable forensic technique that provided admissible scientific evidence in criminal trials. Many cases decided after *Jakobetz* specifically cite the case as a precedent in the field, and many courts have based their own decisions on the reasoning and ruling laid out in the appeals court's ruling. In a broader sense, the court's decision was framed within the context of novel scientific procedures in general (which, at the time, DNA typing was), therefore setting a standard for any new scientific procedure whose admissibility is questioned.

DAUBERT V. MERRELL DOW PHARMACEUTICALS, 509 U.S. 579 (1993)

Background

In the early 1980s in San Diego, two children were born with birth defects. One, Jason Daubert, had only two fingers on his right hand and was missing a bone in his right arm. The other, Eric Schuller, was born without a left hand and with one leg shorter than the other. The mothers of both children had taken the anti-nausea drug Benedictin, produced by Merrell

Dow Pharmaceuticals, during their pregnancies. The parents decided to sue Merrell Dow, claiming that their children's birth defects were a result of the mothers' exposure to Benedictin. At the first trial, Merrell Dow called an expert witness, Dr. Steven H. Lamm, who testified that Benedictin had been subjected to intensive trials with humans, and that no evidence existed for teratogenic effects of the drug in humans. (Teratogenic effects are those that cause malformations in a fetus.) In response, the petitioners called eight witnesses of their own who drew on animal studies and comparisons of the chemical structure of Benedictin to that of other teratogens to conclude that the drug could cause birth defects. These witnesses also testified that they reanalyzed Merrell Dow's original studies with humans and concluded that those studies showed that the drug could have teratogenic effects in humans. The court found for the respondents and dismissed the case. The petitioners appealed, and the case was argued before the U.S. Supreme Court on March 30, 1993.

Legal Issues

The primary issue before the Supreme Court was which of two standards on the admissibility of evidence was predominant in this case. At the time, two standards existed. One was the so-called *Frye* standard, enunciated in the 1923 *Frye v. United States* case dealing with evidence from polygraph testing. In that case, the court had ruled that evidence could be admitted if the technology or procedure on which it was based was generally accepted within the field from which it came. The second standard was one set out in the Federal Rules of Evidence (FRE), adopted in 1975. That standard was somewhat less restrictive. It permitted evidence that has "any tendency to make the existence of any fact that is of consequence to the determination of the action more probable or less probable than it would be without the evidence." In particular, with regard to scientific evidence, it permitted any evidence that "will assist the trier of fact to understand the evidence or to determine a fact in issue."[5]

Decision

The Supreme Court decided that the Federal Rules of Evidence superceded the *Frye* standard and established a new criterion for the admissibility of scientific evidence. It said that such evidence had to meet two standards: (1) reliability and (2) relevance. That is, a judge had to be convinced that a witness appearing before the court was competent to present accurate information that would help the judge and/or a jury to better understand the facts in a case and to make an informed decision based on those facts. The witness also had to be an expert in the field in which he or she was testifying. The Court declared, in a now famous phrase, that the judge was to be a "gatekeeper" of scientific knowledge introduced into a case, determining what information was useful and relevant and what was not. The Court remanded the case to the district court, which again found for the respondents. It decided that the manipulation of earlier human studies by petitioners' experts had not been subjected to scientific scrutiny and, thus, did not meet the Supreme Court's criterion of reliability and relevance.

Impact

The Supreme Court's decision to accept the looser standards established in the Federal Rules of Evidence in preference to the *Frye* standard marked a revolution in judicial philosophy in the United States. It permitted judges a much broader range of options in allowing expert testimony. Some observers have praised this change, arguing that it allows judges and juries to hear a greater range of scientific opinion in making decisions on technical issues. Others have expressed reservations about the more liberal standards, however. They are concerned that these standards will make it easier for experts to present scientific views that have not yet been widely adopted within the scientific community, misleading judges and juries as to what experts in the field actually believe. A number of writers have expressed concern that the looser standards might lead to a flood of cases in which absurd or irrational pseudoscientific ideas might be passed on as accepted facts.

The Supreme Court acknowledged these concerns in its *Daubert* decision and suggested a number of criteria that judges might use in determining the accuracy of scientific information presented in a case. They said that such information (1) should be subject to scientific tests; (2) has been subjected to peer review and publication; (3) has a rate of error that can be estimated; (4) can be compared to generally accepted standards in the field from which it comes; and (5) has been accepted by a significant portion of practitioners in the field of science involved.

In any case, the *Daubert* standard remains the primary criterion on which the admissibility of scientific information in a field is accepted. The standard has been raised recently in a number of cases involving the use of fingerprints as evidence in criminal trials. Defendants have argued that fingerprint evidence does not meet the standards established by *Daubert* and that, therefore, such evidence is not admissible in a court of law. For example, they claim that little or no scientific evidence exists to support that view that all fingerprints are unique and that claims to that effect are based on folklore rather than science. Thus far, so-called *Daubert* challenges to convictions based on fingerprint evidence have not been successful on either state or federal levels.

UNITED STATES V. SCHEFFER, 961133 (1998)

Background

In 1992 Edward Scheffer was serving in the U.S. Army at Marsh Air Force Base in California. He had been asked by the Air Force Office of Special Investigations (OSI) to serve as an OSI undercover agent in certain drug investigations. Scheffer was told that he would be expected to provide urine samples and take polygraph tests as a regular part of this assignment. He accepted the offer and agreed to the testing arrangements. In April 1992, Scheffer went AWOL (absent without leave) from Marsh. Shortly before he was reported absent from his assignment, he had provided a urine sample and volunteered to take a polygraph test. The results of the urinalysis had not become available when he went AWOL. Two weeks later Sheffer was picked up by a local police officer during a routine traffic stop. At that point, he was charged with a number of crimes, including passing bad checks while he was AWOL and having failed his earlier drug test (it had been positive for methamphetamine). As part of his defense in the ensuing trial, Scheffer asked to have his polygraph test admitted in evidence. The polygraph test had showed that he was telling the truth when he told examiners that he had not used drugs since joining the air force.

Scheffer was found guilty of all charges by a military trial judge and sentenced to a bad-conduct discharge, confinement for 30 months in a military stockade, total forfeiture of all pay and allowances, and reduction to the lowest enlisted grade. Upon appeal, the Air Force Court of Criminal Appeals affirmed the trial judge's decision. At the next level of appeal, however, the United States Court of Appeals for the Armed Forces reversed the lower court rulings, arguing that Scheffer's Sixth Amendment right to present a valid defense had been violated. The case then moved one step higher, to the U.S. Supreme Court, which heard arguments on November 3, 1997.

Legal Issues

The Supreme Court was faced with two issues in the Scheffer case. First, does an individual (Scheffer in this case) have the right to present evidence that might tend to support his or her plea of innocence in the case? Second, is evidence obtained from polygraph testing sufficiently reliable to be admissible in a court of law? As it turns out, the two issues are inextricably related.

Decision

Justice Thomas, writing for the Court, explained that a defendant's right to present evidence on his or her behalf is not unlimited. Such evidence must have sufficient relevance to and bearing on a case to make it worthy of a judge's or jury's attention. The inclusion of irrelevant evidence serves only to distract decision makers from the primary issues involved in the case.

In this instance, Thomas wrote, polygraph evidence is not relevant because polygraph testing had still not attained the necessary level of acceptance in the scientific community. "The contentions of respondent and the dissent notwithstanding," Thomas wrote, "there is simply no consensus that polygraph evidence is reliable. To this day, the scientific community remains extremely polarized about the reliability of polygraph techniques."[6] He went on to point out that, although the degree of reliability of polygraph evidence depends on a variety of factors, "there is simply no way to know in a particular case whether a polygraph examiner's conclusion is accurate, because certain doubts and uncertainties plague even the best polygraph exams." As a result, he noted, decisions about the admissibility of polygraph evidence have varied widely across federal and state jurisdictions. Lacking any consistent scientific validation, the Court ruled, polygraph testing is still inadmissible in courts of law. Since such evidence is inadmissible, then a defendant has no constitutional right to ask that it be used in a trial.

Impact

A decade later, the argument presented in *United States v. Scheffer* remains the standard in U.S. courts. Clarified by the highest court's position on the issue, lower courts have consistently ruled that polygraph testing has not yet reached a stage of scientific acceptance that its results can be admitted in courts of law.

KUMHO TIRE CO. V. CARMICHAEL, 526 U.S. 137 (1999)

Background

On July 6, 1993, in Montgomery, Alabama, a tire on a vehicle driven by Patrick Carmichael blew out, causing the vehicle to overturn. One passenger was killed in the accident and the remaining passengers were injured. The decedent's survivors and the injured passengers brought suit against Kumho Tire, makers of the damaged tire, claiming that the product was defective. They offered in evidence the expert testimony of Dennis Carlson, Jr., a tire failure analyst. Carlson testified that his investigation of the damaged tire indicated that it had been improperly made and the accident was a result of this. Kumho moved to exclude Carlson's testimony on the basis that it did not meet existing standards of admissibility, specifically Federal Rule of Evidence (FRE) 702 and the criteria established by the Supreme Court in *Daubert v. Merrell Dow Pharmaceuticals, Inc.* The district court allowed Kumho's motion, stating that Carlson's testimony had met none of the criteria established by *Daubert*. Upon appeal, the Eleventh Circuit Court reversed the district court's decision, writing that it had improperly applied *Daubert* standards since Carlson was not a scientist and, hence, not covered by the *Daubert* ruling. The case was then appealed to the U.S. Supreme Court.

Legal Issues

The single issue with which the Supreme Court had to deal was whether the circuit court was correct in excluding Carlson's testimony because he was an engineer and not a scientist and, hence, not covered by the Court's earlier *Daubert* ruling and the standards for admissibility of evidence created by that case. The circuit court specifically referred to an earlier ruling by the Sixth Circuit Court that had written that "the distinction between scientific and nonscientific expert testimony is a critical one." Following that reasoning, the Eleventh Circuit Court reversed the decision of the district court.

Decision

The Supreme Court ruled that the Eleventh Circuit Court (and, by implication, the Sixth Circuit Court) had erred in limiting its *Daubert* standards to scientific testimony. It explained that the four criteria established in *Daubert* had referred to scientists because the case at hand (*Daubert v. Merrell Dow*) had dealt with scientific issues. The Court pointed out that the relevant Federal Rules of Evidence (702 and 703) "grant all expert witnesses, not just 'scientific' ones, testimonial latitude unavailable to other witnesses on the assumption that the expert's opinion will have a reliable basis in the knowledge and experience of his discipline." Finally, the Court pointed out the practical difficulty faced by courts in distinguishing between expert testimony that is scientific and non-scientific because, in general, "there is no clear line dividing the one from the others and no convincing need to make such distinctions."[7] In a unanimous decision, the Court reversed the Eleventh Circuit Court's opinion.

Impact

Kumho is an important decision because it eliminated a loophole frequently used by attorneys to avoid having to deal with *Daubert* standards. In cases where they wished to introduce "expert" testimony, they could argue that the testimony was not "scientific," and, therefore, not subject to the strict standards required by *Daubert*. What the Supreme Court said in *Kumho* was that it didn't make any difference whether "expert" testimony was scientific or not, as long as it was truly specialized knowledge that only an expert in the field could supply. In such cases, the standards set by *Daubert* applied and a *Daubert* hearing was required if requested.

UNITED STATES OF AMERICA V. BYRON C. MITCHELL, CRIMINAL CASE NO. 9600407 (1999)

Background

In 1991, Byron Mitchell was charged with armed robbery in Philadelphia. Among the evidence presented at his trial were an anonymous note identifying a vehicle used in the commission of the crime and a set of fingerprints identified as belonging to Mitchell. The trial judge admitted both pieces of evidence, and at least partly on the basis of this evidence, Mitchell was convicted of the crime. He was sentenced to 24 years in prison and restitution of $19,100 of the $20,000 stolen in the robbery. On appeal, the trial court's decision was reversed on the basis of improper admission of the anonymous note. Just prior to retrial of the case in 1998, the defense submitted a one-page notice of intention to file a request for a *Daubert* hearing. *Daubert* hearings are based on the famous *Daubert v. Merrell Dow Pharmaceuticals* case of 1993 in which standards for the admission of scientific evidence and scientific testimony were established. The defense proposed to offer testimony from an expert witness, James E. Starrs, professor of law and forensic science at George Washington University Law School, to the effect that no scientific evidence exists for the claim of the uniqueness of fingerprints.

Legal Issues

Lacking admissibility of the anonymous note identifying a vehicle used in the 1991 Philadelphia robbery, the reprosecution of Byron Mitchell rested most heavily on a set of fingerprints obtained at the scene of the crime and identified by experts as belonging to the defendant. Since the 1911 case of *People v. Jennings*, fingerprint evidence had been routinely accepted as evidence in court cases at every jurisdictional level, from local to federal, without question as to its scientific validity. *United States v. Mitchell* was the first case in which a defendant had raised the possibility that fingerprints are not unique and that, therefore, they cannot be used as a means of identification in criminal cases. At Mitchell's retrial, the court was faced with two major issues. First, does sufficient scientific evidence for the individuality of fingerprints exist to permit the admission of prints as evidence in criminal cases? The prosecution actually asked the court to confirm the scientific status of fingerprints, in general, and, hence, their admissibility in criminal cases. Second, should professor Starrs (and/or other experts in the field) be allowed to appear as a witness for the defense?

Decision

The court's decision, presented orally on September 13, 1999, provided a mixed message for the legal community. On the one hand, the presiding judge declined to allow Starrs and other defense witnesses to testify on the scientific validity of fingerprinting. Those witnesses could conceivably have testified on other aspects of the case, such as the match between fingerprints found at the scene and those obtained from Mitchell. But the defense did not offer the witnesses for any purpose other than questioning the scientific validity of fingerprints. On the other hand, the judge declined to act on the government's request to declare the scientific validity of fingerprinting. Instead, he ruled that the question was irrelevant to the case at hand. What mattered was that the fingerprint evidence submitted did provide useful information on the case and, on that basis alone it could legitimately be admitted in evidence.

Impact

The law enforcement and legal communities have been somewhat concerned about possible successful challenges to the use of fingerprint evidence. Such evidence has been used successfully in thousands of criminal cases over the past century. Still, critics are correct in noting that very little hard scientific evidence exists to support the contention that fingerprints are unique. Challenges to the validity of fingerprint evidence have continued following *United States v. Mitchell*, but almost none of them has been successful. In 2002, U.S. District Judge Louis Pollak became the first jurist to accept the arguments of antifingerprint experts and excluded such evidence in a Philadelphia murder trial. Pollak's decision greatly troubled lawyers and police officers, but their concerns lasted only a short time. Only a few weeks after issuing his decision, Pollak changed his mind and agreed to admit the fingerprint evidence he had previously banned. Most fingerprint experts believe, however, that tests of the validity of fingerprint evidence will continue to be offered in the future, at least one of which may someday survive judicial review.

---

[1] Federal Rules of Evidence. Available online. URL: http://www.law.cornell.edu/rules/fre/. Accessed on July 3, 2007.

[2] Quoted in Mark A. Acree, "*People v. Jennings:* A Significant Case in American Fingerprint History." Available online. URL: http://www.scafo.org/library/140401.html. Accessed on July 6, 2007.

[3] Quoted in Darrell Klasey, "*State v. Kuhl* and the California Connection," *The California Identification Digest*, vol. 6, no. 4, July/August 2006, p. 14.

[4] *United States v. Jakobetz*, 955 F.2d 786 (2nd Cir. 01/09/1992). Available online. URL: http://www.cjcentral.com/jakobetz.htm. Accessed on July 6, 2007.

[5] *Daubert v. Merrell Dow Pharmaceuticals, Inc.*, 509 U.S. 579 (1993). Available online. URL: http://caselaw.lp.findlaw.com/scripts/getcase.pl?court=US&vol=509&invol=579. Accessed on July 6, 2007.

[6] *United States v. Scheffer* (96-1133), 44 M. J. 442, reversed. Available online. URL: http://www.law.cornell.edu/supct/html/96-1133.ZO.html. Accessed on July 6, 2007.

[7] *Kumho Tire Co. v. Carmichael* (97-1709), 526 U.S. 137 (1999), 131 F.3d 1433, reversed. Available online. URL: http://supct.la.cornell.edu.supct/html/97-1709.ZO.html. Accessed on July 6, 2007.

CHAPTER 3

CHRONOLOGY

This chapter presents a chronology of major events in the history of the development of new technologies in forensic sciences, including scientific and technological advances, as well as political, social, ethical, and other events related to forensic research.

ABOUT A.D. 700

- Chinese business documents and divorce decrees contain fingerprints that have been affixed for purposes of identification, although no specific system has been developed for classifying the prints.

1ST CENTURY

- The Roman lawyer Quintilian shows that bloody palm prints have been used in an attempt to frame a blind man for the murder of his mother.

14TH CENTURY

- Official government documents from the Persian government contain fingerprints that appear to be used for purposes of identification.

1537

- Italian mathematician Niccolò Tartaglia publishes "Nova scientia," a work in which he discusses characteristic markings left by the firing of a gun.

1686

- Marcello Malpighi, professor of anatomy at the University of Bologna, describes the pattern of ridges found on fingertips, but makes no connection between his discoveries and their possible applications to forensic science.

Chronology

1730

- English writer Daniel Defoe suggests taking the pulse of a suspected criminal as a way of determining his or her possible guilt or innocence in a crime.

1794

- ***March 23:*** 18-year-old John Toms is convicted of the murder of Edward Culshaw in Prescot, Lancashire, England. It is believed to be the first criminal case in which ballistic evidence is used to obtain a conviction.

1818

- English naturalist Thomas Bewick uses engravings of his own fingerprints to identify books he has published.

1823

- Jan Evangelista Purkinje, professor of anatomy at the University of Breslau, publishes the first scientific paper on the classification of fingerprints.

1835

- Belgian social scientist and statistician Adolphe Quételet publishes *Sur l'homme et le développement de ses facultés* (*A Treatise on Man, and the Development of His Faculties*), in which he outlines the principles of a statistical analysis of human physical characteristics.
- A London police officer, Henry Goddard, compares the markings on a bullet used in a murder to the mold from which it came, thereby identifying the person responsible for the crime.

1838

- One William Stewart, of Baltimore, is convicted of murdering his father based on ballistic evidence obtained from an analysis of bullets found at the scene of the crime and bullets belonging to the suspect's gun. It is the first case in the United States in which a conviction is obtained on the basis of ballistic evidence.

1854

- ***March 27:*** One R. V. Richardson of Lincoln, England, is convicted of the murder of a policeman based on the discovery that paper fragments found at the scene of the crime match those used as a firing wad in the pistol owned by Richardson.

1858

- Sir William Herschel, an officer in the Indian Civil Service, initiates the practice of using thumbprints as a substitute for written signatures on official documents verified by illiterate workers.

1876

- Italian criminologist Cesare Lombroso publishes *L'Uomo delinquente (Criminal man)*, in which he outlines his theory that criminals can be recognized by certain characteristic physiological features.
- In what may be the first court ruling of its kind, a state court in Georgia permits a firearms expert to testify about ballistic evidence regarding the time passed since a bullet had been fired in a crime.

1878

- Italian physiologist Angelo Mosso reports on the use of an instrument he calls the plethysmograph, which measures a person's breath rate and blood flow.

1880

- ***October 8:*** Scottish physician Henry Faulds publishes a paper in the journal *Nature* describing the use of fingerprints to exonerate a person of a crime in Tokyo, Japan. He suggests that fingerprinting may have widespread use in forensic science for the solving of crimes.

1883

- French anthropologist and criminology Alphonse Bertillon introduces the practice of identifying "criminal types" on the basis of certain body measurements.

1884

- Francis Galton establishes an anthropometric laboratory for the purpose of collecting physical data, including fingerprint data, on a large number of individuals for possible use in identification procedures.

1888

- Alphonse Bertillon is appointed chief of the newly created Department of Judicial Identity at the Paris Préfecture.
- Austrian jurist and criminologist Hans Gross publishes one of the first great books on criminology, *Criminal Investigation*, in which he recommends the use of anthropometry in the identification of criminals.

Chronology

1889

- French criminologist Alexandre Lacassagne publishes "La Deformation des Balles de Revolver" ("Deformation of Revolver Bullets") in the journal *Archive de Anthropologie criminelle et des Sciences Pénales*, describing the process by which bullets fired from a gun leave characteristic markings on the gun barrel.

1892

- English polymath Sir Francis Galton publishes *Fingerprints*, his first extensive work on the use of fingerprinting as a tool of identification, in which he attempts to estimate the mathematical probability of two different individuals having the same set of fingerprints.
- Juan Vucetich, Croatian-Argentinian anthropologist and criminologist, develops the first scientific system for classifying fingerprints.

1895

- Italian criminologist Cesare Lombroso publishes research papers in which he describes the use of Mosso's plethysmograph in the interrogation of criminal suspects.

1896

- Sir Edward Henry, then head of the Metropolitan Police of London, publishes *Classification and Uses of Finger Prints*, a book that contains a system for classifying fingerprints that becomes the standard in Europe and North America.
- Argentina becomes one of the first nations in the world to adopt fingerprinting, in preference to anthropometry, for criminal identification.

1897

- ***June 12:*** The British governor-general of India orders that fingerprinting be used instead of anthropometry for the identification of criminals in the areas under his command on the Indian subcontinent.

1898

- German forensic chemist Paul Jesrich conducts the first microscopic examination and comparison of markings left by bullets fired from a gun.

1900

- ***June:*** Dr. Albert Llewellyn Hall publishes the first scholarly article on ballistic analysis, "The Missile and the Weapon," in the *Buffalo Medical Journal.*

1901

- ***July 1:*** The first fingerprint department in England is established at Scotland Yard, under the direction of Sir Edward Richard Henry.

1902

- ***September 13:*** A burglar by the name of Henry Jackson is the first person in the United Kingdom convicted on the basis of fingerprint evidence.
- ***October 24:*** Alphonse Bertillon makes the first criminal identification of a fingerprint without a known suspect.

1903

- ***May 4:*** In one of the classic cases in forensic identification in the United States, a criminal suspect by the name of Will West is identified at Leavenworth Penitentiary in Kansas by his fingerprints, after efforts to make an identification by means of anthropometry proved to be unsuccessful.

1905

- The U.S. Army initiates the practice of fingerprinting all of its service members.
- The U.S. Department of Justice (DOJ) creates a Bureau of Criminal Identification (BCI) responsible for creating a centralized database of fingerprints.
- ***May:*** Fingerprints are used for the first time in a murder trial in Great Britain at the trial of Alfred and Albert Stratton, who are found guilty of murdering a shopkeeper by the name of Ann Farrow.

1908

- ***July 26:*** U.S. Attorney General Charles Bonaparte appoints a group of ten special agents within the Department of Justice (DOJ) to investigate federal crimes, which eventually is named the Bureau of Investigation (BI). The bureau is the earliest predecessor of the modern day Federal Bureau of Investigation (FBI).

1911

- ***February 1:*** In the case of *People v. Jennings*, defendant Thomas Jennings becomes the first person in the United States to be convicted of murder on the basis of fingerprint evidence.

Chronology

1912

- French criminologist Edmond Locard publishes his classic seven-volume work *Traité de criminalistique (Treaty on Criminalistics)*, which details his system of porosity, in which the pore patterns in a person's fingerprints can be used for the identification of individuals.

1913

- Victor Balthazard, professor of forensic medicine at the Sorbonne, in Paris, publishes the first article on the unique characteristics of markings on bullets.
- ***March:*** Italian psychologist Vittorio Benussi presents a paper before the Italian Society for Psychology (ISP) in Rome, describing his experiments on the correlations between lying and three physical traits: respiration rate, pulse rate, and blood pressure.

1914

- ***February 13:*** The science of anthropometric analysis for the purpose of criminal identifications dies out rapidly with the death of its founder and principal advocate, Alphonse Bertillon.

1916

- The government of Argentina creates the General Register of Identification, requiring all citizens of the country to be fingerprinted.

1917

- William Moulton Marston, then a student at Harvard Law School, publishes his first reports on a lie detector machine on which he has been working for five years.

1918

- ***September 5:*** In the case of *State v. Kuhl*, the Nevada Supreme Court upholds a lower court decision based on palm prints of the defendant, the first state supreme court to admit palm prints as valid evidence in criminal trials in the state.

1921

- John Larson, a psychologist employed by the Berkeley (California) Police Department invents a device for making continuous records of a person's respiration rate and heart beat.

- J. H. Taylor, chief of identification for the U.S. Navy, devises a system for identifying individuals on the basis of a single fingerprint, in contrast to all previous fingerprint systems, which rely on a complete set of ten fingerprints.

1922

- Paul V. Hadley is convicted in Arizona of the murder of a couple from whom he hitched a ride outside Tucson. His conviction is achieved to a large extent because of an exhaustive study of ballistic evidence collected at the scene of the crime. Upon appeal, the Arizona Supreme Court upholds the decision, making it the first state supreme court in the United States to explicitly confirm the admissibility of ballistic evidence.

1923

- In the first recorded use of polygraph testing on behalf of a commercial business, John Larson tests 38 coeds at the University of California in an effort to identify a shoplifter at a local store. The test results in admission of guilt by one employee.
- The comparison microscope is developed by photographer Philip O. Gravelle. The microscope allows one to compare markings on two bullets at the same time.
- ***December 3:*** In *Frye v. United States*, the federal court of appeals for the District of Columbia rules that polygraph testing has not yet reached sufficient standing within the scientific community for its results to be accepted in legal disputes.

1924

- ***July 1:*** The Identification Division is created as part of the Federal Bureau of Investigation (FBI). The division becomes the central repository for both the collection of fingerprints then held at the Leavenworth Penitentiary in Kansas and similar collections held by more than 5,000 law enforcement agencies throughout the United States.

1925

- ***April:*** C. E. Waite, Calvin H. Goddard, Philip O. Gravelle, and John H. Fisher establish the Bureau of Forensic Ballistics in New York City for the purpose of providing firearms identification services for forensic scientists throughout the United States.
- ***November–December:*** Calvin H. Goddard coins the term *forensic ballistics* in an article, " Forensic Ballistics," published in the November–December issue of the magazine *Army Ordnance*.

Chronology

1926

- Leonard Keeler, a protégé of John Larson, improves Larson's polygraph machine by adding a system for measuring galvanic skin reflex changes.

1928

- New York becomes the first state to adopt a law mandating the fingerprinting of all individuals arrested and charged with a misdemeanor or felony.

1929

- ***June:*** The first true national crime laboratory, the Scientific Crime Detection Laboratory (SCDL), is established in Chicago, Illinois, largely in response to the St. Valentine's Day massacre. Within a short period of time the SCDL became affiliated with Northwestern University in nearby Evanston.

1930

- ***January:*** The staff at the Scientific Crime Detection Laboratory (SCDL) in Chicago, Illinois, founds the nation's first forensic journal, the *American Journal of Police Science*. The journal is later absorbed by the *Journal of Criminal Law and Criminology* and renamed the *Journal of Criminal Law, Criminology, and Police Science*.

1938

- E. Patrick Coffey, special agent for the Federal Bureau of Investigation (FBI), becomes the agency's first official polygraphist and uses the lie detector in an espionage investigation for the first time in the United States.
- The Scientific Crime Detection Laboratory (SCDL) is purchased by the city of Chicago, Illinois, from Northwestern University and moved from the Northwestern campus to downtown Chicago. The laboratory remains the premier center for forensic research in the United States.

1948

- Leonard Keeler, John Reid, and Fred Inbau open the first school designed to train polygraph operators—the Keeler Institute, in Chicago, Illinois.
- ***January 19–21:*** The American Academy of Forensic Science (AAFS) is established at a meeting of forensic scientists and others interested in criminology in St. Louis, Missouri. The initial meeting of the organization is

called the First American Medicolegal Congress, and the organization's formal name is not adopted until 1950.

1951

- The U.S. Army establishes the U.S. Army Polygraph School (USAPI) as part of the Provost Marshal General School at Fort Gordon, Georgia. USAPI is redesignated as the Department of Defense Polygraph Institute (DoDPI) in 1985.

1969

- ***February:*** The Association of Firearm and Toolmark Examiners (AFTE) is formed in Chicago, Illinois, under the auspices of the American Academy of Forensic Science (AAFS) and the Chicago Police Department.

1971

- ***November 29:*** The U.S. National Crime Information Center (NCIC) adds to its database a Computerized Criminal History (CCH) file containing detailed descriptions of individuals arrested for serious crimes. The CCH includes a computerized fingerprint classification and identification system.

1975

- ***January 2:*** The U.S. Congress agrees to the adoption of the Federal Rules of Evidence (FRE), the first national set of standards for the admissibility of documents, testimony, reports, and other materials in federal trials.

1977

- The Federal Bureau of Investigation (FBI) begins using an Automated Fingerprint Identification System (AFIS) to create computerized scans of fingerprints.
- ***May:*** Fuseo Matsumura, an employee at the Saga Prefectural Crime Laboratory of the National Police Agency in Japan, accidentally discovers a method for developing latent fingerprints by using a commercial product known as superglue.

1980

- The Federal Bureau of Investigation (FBI) initiates a program for sharing its General Rifling Characteristics (GRC) file with law enforcement agencies and forensic laboratories throughout the United States, as part of its National Crime Information Center.

Chronology

1983

- Kerry Mullis develops the polymerase chain reaction (PCR), a method for replicating small samples of DNA so that they can be used for, among other applications, forensic analysis.

1984

- Sir Alec Jeffreys develops a process known as restriction fragment length polymorphism (RFLP), a technique by which the DNA from different organisms can be distinguished from each other.

1986

- Forensic scientists use DNA typing to exonerate a suspect in the murder of two girls in England. The procedure is also used in obtaining the conviction of Colin Pitchfork, the person who actually committed the crime. The case is the first one in which DNA typing is used to solve a crime.
- Henry Ehrlich and his colleagues at the Cetus Corporation develop the first commercially available DNA typing kit for use in forensic studies of crimes.
- ***December:*** Edward Blake, a consultant in forensic biology, uses DNA typing in the case of *People v. Pestinikas* to confirm that defendants in the case, owners of a nursing home, had not switched organs of an elderly man who had died at their facility. The Pestinikas are convicted of homicide in the case, however. The case is the first instance in which DNA typing is accepted by a civil court in the United States.

1988

- The Federal Bureau of Investigation (FBI) establishes its own laboratory for the testing of DNA samples in criminal investigations.
- ***February 6:*** Orlando, Florida, resident Tommy Lee Andrews is convicted of rape, at least partly as the result of DNA evidence submitted by the prosecution. The case is the first instance in the United States in which DNA typing is accepted in a criminal case.
- ***June 27:*** President Ronald Reagan signs the Employee Polygraph Protection Act of 1988, which prohibits, with certain exceptions, employers from using lie detector tests for either preemployment screening or during the course of employment.

1989

- ***August 14:*** The admissibility of DNA typing evidence is challenged for the first time in the United States in the case of *People v. Castro*. The court rules that DNA typing can be used to exclude suspects, but not as evidence of the guilt of a suspect.

- ***September:*** In the case of *Spencer v. Commonwealth*, the Virginia Supreme Court confirms the death penalty for Timothy Wilson based on DNA evidence found on the bodies of several victims. The case is the first instance in which DNA evidence results in the death penalty for a convicted felon.

1990

- The Federal Bureau of Investigation (FBI) introduces the Combined DNA Index System (CODIS) on a pilot basis. The system is designed to provide an efficient mechanism by which state, local, and national law enforcement agencies and forensic laboratories can exchange information with each other.

1991

- ***June 27:*** President George H. W. Bush promulgates Military Rule of Evidence (MRE) 707, which prohibits the use of results obtained from polygraph testing in any military trial.

1992

- ***April 14:*** A special committee of the National Research Council of the National Academy of Sciences publishes a report on the use of DNA typing in forensic science. The report is entitled *DNA Technology and Forensic Science*.
- ***July:*** The Federal Bureau of Investigation (FBI) installs a new electronic database and computer network called DRUGFIRE that stores and links unique markings left on bullets and shell casings after a gun is fired.

1993

- ***June 28:*** In the case of *Daubert v. Merrell Dow*, the U.S. Supreme Court for the first time in 70 years changes the standards for determining the admissibility of evidence offered by expert witnesses.

1994

- ***September 13:*** The U.S. Congress passes a set of amendments to the Omnibus Crime Control and Safe Streets Act of 1968 that includes three sections concerned with DNA testing.

1995

- ***April:*** The United Kingdom National Criminal Intelligence DNA Database (NDNAD) is established as part of the Forensic Science Service of the Home Office. As of 2006, NDNAD held information on about 3.5 million individuals.

1996

- ***December:*** The National Research Council of the National Academy of Sciences publishes a report, *The Evaluation of Forensic DNA Evidence*, providing an extensive review of the scientific and legal status of DNA typing and outlining recommended procedures for use of the technique in criminal cases.

1998

- ***March 31:*** In *U.S. v. Scheffer*, the U.S. Supreme Court rules that disallowing the submission of polygraph test results by a defendant is not a violation of the defendant's Fifth and Sixth Amendment right to present an adequate defense.
- ***October 13:*** The Federal Bureau of Investigation (FBI) announces the introduction of its new National DNA Index System (NDIS). NDIS is the highest level of the Combined DNA Index System (CODIS) that allows law enforcement agencies and forensic science laboratories to exchange information about serial violent crimes and sex offenders.

1999

- ***January 29:*** The Federal Bureau of Investigation (FBI) introduces a computerized fingerprint classification and identification system called the Integrated Automatic Fingerprint Identification System (IAFIS) capable of holding 65 million records.
- ***July 7–13:*** The first major challenge to fingerprint evidence in U.S. courts is presented at a case heard before the United States Court of Appeals for the Third Circuit in the case *of United States of America v. Byron Mitchell.*

2003

- ***March 11:*** Attorney General John Ashcroft announces creation of the President's DNA Initiative, a program to provide funding, training, and assistance of federal, state, and local forensic laboratories and law enforcement personnel with the goal of ensuring that DNA typing is used to its greatest potential in solving crimes, protecting the innocent, and identifying missing persons.

2004

- ***November 2:*** Voters in California adopt Proposition 69 requiring that DNA fingerprints be taken from everyone arrested for or charged with a felony.

2005

- ***July 15:*** Attorney Brandon Mayfield files suit in U.S. District Court after he had been arrested as a suspect in the 2004 Madrid train bombings based on a supposed fingerprint match with prints taken from the crime scene. The fingerprint match later turned out to be erroneous.

2006

- ***January 5:*** President George W. Bush signs the 2005 Violence Against Women Act and the 2005 Department of Justice (DOJ) Reauthorization Act, both of which contain portions of earlier legislation (the DNA Fingerprinting Act) extending DNA legislation to cover certain illegal aliens.

2007

- ***April 2:*** Researchers Charles R. Honts and Susan Amato publish a study indicating that automated polygraph testing may produce more accurate results than tests conducted by humans.
- ***April 4:*** The Taunton, Massachusetts, school committee announces that students will be able to purchase their lunches by "signing" for them with their fingerprints.
- ***August 1:*** Researchers at the Department of Chemical Engineering, Imperial College London, and the Home Office Scientific Development Branch in the United Kingdom announce that they had found a method for analyzing the chemical composition of fingerprints, allowing a more complete and detailed analysis of prints left at a crime scene.
- ***October 13:*** California governor Arnold Schwarzenegger signs legislation requiring "microstamping" by 2010 of all new semiautomatic handgun models sold in California. The legislation requires that every cartridge fired from certain types of guns carry a distinctive code that will identify the weapon and ammunition.
- ***November 16:*** Researchers at the Indian Institute of Technology in New Delhi announce that they have developed a system for scanning fingerprints with optical coherence tomography, a laser-like system for reading ridges and grooves. The new system permits the reading and analysis of fingerprints without using dusting or other traditional methods.

2008

- ***January 1:*** Fingerprint requirements are an important part of a number of new laws in the state of Texas, including a requirement that anyone applying for a new or renewed broker's or salesperson's license submit his or her fingerprints to the the state.

- ***January 1:*** Japan introduces a new program for the fingerprinting of the vast majority of individuals entering the country.
- ***January 14:*** The British government announces that its new program requiring everyone who enters the country to be fingerprinted has already uncovered more than 500 illegal immigrants.

CHAPTER 4

BIOGRAPHICAL LISTING

This chapter contains brief biographical sketches of individuals who have played major roles in the development of fingerprint analysis, ballistic analysis, anthropometry, polygraph testing, and DNA typing or who have made contributions to related aspects of these fields.

Tommy Lee Andrews, the first person in the United States to have been convicted of a crime based on evidence obtained from DNA typing. In February 1987, warehouse worker Tommy Lee Andrews broke into the home of a 27-year-old woman and raped and assaulted her repeatedly. The woman claimed to have had a good look at her assailant and was able to pick Andrews out of a lineup held by local investigators. Fingerprints and blood samples taken from the crime scene also matched samples provided by Andrews, although the match in both cases was not very good. Having just heard of the success of DNA typing in solving the Colin Pitchfork case in England, prosecutors hired Lifecodes, a laboratory in Valhalla, New York, to conduct DNA tests of evidence found at the crime scene and a blood sample provided by Andrews. A Lifecodes scientist concluded that the likelihood of an erroneous match in this case was one in 10 billion. Defense lawyers forced the scientist to recant on this testimony, but two weeks later he repeated his evidence, with sufficient scientific support to validate his calculations. Based largely on the DNA evidence, Andrews was convicted of rape and aggravated assault and sentenced to 22 years in prison.

David R. Ashbaugh, staff sergeant (retired) of the Royal Canadian Mounted Police (RCMP). Ashbaugh is one of the world's authorities on the analysis of digital fingerprints. He was on active duty for 36 years with the RCMP, 28 of which he was a Certified Forensic Identification Specialist. He has conducted extensive research on the scientific basis of digital fingerprinting and has suggested the term *ridgeology* for the most up-to-date, scientifically based system of identifying fingerprints. He is author of *Quantitative-Qualitative Friction Ridge Analysis*, widely acknowledged as the standard work in the field of digital fingerprinting.

William Joseph Babler, associate professor at the Indiana University School of Dentistry. He is an expert in the prenatal development of human fingerprints. Although Babler's primary field of research interest is in craniofacial growth and craniofacial morphology, he has carried out groundbreaking research in the way that fingerprint patterns develop prior to birth. His studies have showed that fingerprint patterns are developed from volar pads that first appear about six weeks after fertilization in the growing embryo: High volar pads develop into whorls, while low volar pads develop into arches.

Victor Balthazard, professor of forensic medicine at the Sorbonne and chief medical officer with the French Sûreté during the early decades of the 20th century. Early in his career, Balthazard worked on the medical applications of radiation with Pierre Curie in Paris and introduced the concept of using bismuth compounds for stomach X-rays. He later became interested in the forensic applications of medicine and made a number of important breakthroughs in the field. For example, he conducted some of the earliest research on bloodstain analysis, in which the pattern of blood found at a crime scene is analyzed to determine evidence such as the direction from which shots are fired. He also carried out pioneer research on hair samples as evidence at crime scenes and showed, for the first time, how human and animal hair can be distinguished from each other. In 1912, Balthazard gave an address before the Congress of Legal Medicine at which he described his research on the identification of weapons from which bullets are fired. That address and a later article, the first of its kind in forensic history, led to the acceptance of ballistic analysis as a fruitful and legitimate specialty in the field of forensic science.

Vittorio Benussi, Italian psychologist and philosopher who developed an instrument for measuring a person's rate of respiration, which he pointed out could be used to detect when a person is lying or telling the truth. Benussi's discovery of the relationship between respiration rate and lying constitutes one of the four principal functions of the modern polygraph, the others being pulse rate, blood pressure, and galvanic skin response. Benussi became interested in psychology in his early college years, but took his degree in philosophy because no formal training in psychology was then available (1890s) in Italy. Benussi worked for nearly two decades in Graz, Austria, as a laboratory assistant in psychology, part-time librarian, and freelance researcher. He eventually became a tenured lecturer in experimental psychology at the University of Padua in 1919, where he remained until his death by suicide in 1927.

Alphonse Bertillon, founder of the forensic science of anthropometry, the use of physical measurements of the human body for the identification of criminals. While working as a records clerk at the Paris Sûreté (the French police department), Bertillon decided that the existing system for identifying possible suspects in a crime was much too disorganized to be efficient. He decided to look for ways in which the physical characteristics of an individual—characteristics such as height, weight, the presence of scars and other markings, and features of the eyes and ears—might be correlated with his or her criminal tendencies. At first, Bertillon met with incredulity and derision by members of the police force, and he was forced to conduct his research on his own time. Eventually, however, Bertillon's system led to the identification and conviction of a number of criminals, and it was adopted both in France and in other countries of the world. The system, eventually known as bertillonage in his honor, contained a number of fundamental flaws, however, and it was soon replaced by another means of identification—fingerprinting—that was being developed at about the same time.

Thomas Bewick, sometimes called the father of English book illustration. Bewick's reputation as an engraver of the first order was made with the publication in 1785 of his book, *A General History of Quadrupeds*, although he is equally well known for his brilliant work on the two-volume *History of British Birds* (1797, 1804). To historians of forensic science, Bewick's importance is a consequence of his decision to use his own thumbprint as a unique identifying characteristic on most of his works, not a profound invention, but probably the first of its kind in history.

Govert Bidloo (Govard Bidloo), a late 17th/early 18th-century Dutch anatomist, physician, and playwright. In 1685, Bidloo published an anatomical text, *Anatomia Humani Corporis* (*Anatomy of the Human Body*) that included 105 plates by the artist Gerard de Lairesse, showing detailed studies of various parts of the human body. Among the plates are the first reasonably accurate representations of fingerprint patterns and pores. Much of Bidloo's work was later plagiarized by the English surgeon William Cowper in his own text, *Anatomy of the Human Bodies* (1698).

Simon A. Cole, one of the foremost critics of the use of fingerprinting for individualization in the world today. Cole is currently associate professor in the School of Social Ecology at the University of California at Irvine, where he teaches courses in forensic science and society, surveillance and society, and science, technology, and law. He is probably best known for his book *Suspect Identities: A History of Fingerprinting and Criminal Identification* (Harvard University Press, 2001), which received the 2003 Rachel Carson Prize of the Society for Social Studies of Science. The book provides an excellent review of the methods used by forensic scientists for individualization over the years with an analysis of some problems inherent in the use of those technologies.

Henry Pelouze DeForest, surgeon and obstetrician who worked with the New York Police Department (NYPD) from 1902 to 1912. DeForest received his undergraduate degree from Cornell University and his M.D. from Columbia University in 1884. While serving as a surgeon for the NYPD, DeForest was asked to deal with a problem related to the testing of applicants for civil service positions with the city. In many cases, an applicant might hire a person with more educational background to take the civil service examination in his or her name. The person offered the job, then, was not the same individual who took the examination, resulting in the hiring of many unqualified persons. DeForest developed a system by which applicants taking the civil service examination were fingerprinted, and those prints were then compared with individuals actually offered jobs. The fingerprinting system devised by DeForest is said to have been the first such program of its kind implemented in the United States. DeForest also served as examiner for the New York City Civil Service Commission from 1912 to 1919, as president of the medical board of the Teachers Retirement System from 1917 to 1928, and as professor of obstetrics at the New York Post-Graduate Hospital and Medical School from 1903 to 1921. He is sometimes credited with having invented the dactyloscope, an instrument for comparing fingerprints.

Gary Dotson, the first American to have been exonerated of a crime for which he had been convicted, based on DNA typing evidence. Dotson had been accused in 1977 of raping and kidnaping 16-year-old Cathleen Crowell. He was tried and found guilty in May 1979 and sentenced to 25 to 50 years imprisonment on each count. The conviction was upheld by an appeals court two years later. In 1985, Crowell confessed to her minister that she had lied about the crime, fearing that she had become pregnant as a result of consensual sex with her boyfriend at the time. At a hearing called to reconsider the case, the presiding judge ruled Crowell's recantation less credible than her original testimony. He returned Dotson to prison. Shortly thereafter, Illinois governor James Thompson commuted Dotson's sentence to time served, and he was released from prison. Two years later, he was arrested on a charge of domestic violence, his parole was revoked, and he was returned to prison yet again. Finally, on August 15, 1988, DNA typing results provided positive proof that Dotson was not guilty of the crime for which he had been convicted and one year later he was finally released from prison for good.

Henry Faulds, a Scottish physician and missionary who served in Japan from 1873 to 1886. While serving as superintendent of the Tsukiji Hospital in Tokyo, Faulds visited an archaeological site with a friend and noticed the presence of handprints on ancient pieces of pottery. He began to think about the nature of hand- and fingerprints and came to the conclusion that such prints might be unique for each individual. For this reason, the prints could be used, he decided, for the identification of specific individuals. His theory was put to a test shortly thereafter when a break-in occurred at the hospital. Matching the prints of a suspect arrested by Tokyo police with prints left at the scene of the crime, Faulds was able to prove that the suspect was innocent of the crime. Encouraged by this result, Faulds attempted to interest other scientists in his research. He wrote Charles Darwin, who was too old to take up a study of fingerprints, but passed Faulds's letter to his cousin, Francis Galton. Galton had become interested in fingerprint characteristics himself and was apparently pleased to have Faulds's letter. He, however, never responded to that letter. In November 1880, Faulds published a report of his research in the journal *Nature*, apparently the first written scientific communication on the subject of fingerprinting as a tool for identification. After returning to Great Britain in 1886, Faulds offered his ideas for fingerprinting as a way of identifying criminals to Scotland Yard, which apparently took no action on his suggestions. Losing interest in the effort, Faulds took a job as police surgeon in the town of Fenton in Stoke-on-Trent, where he remained until his death in 1930.

Francis Galton, a Victorian polymath with expertise in a wide variety of fields, including anthropology, statistics, geography, genetics, meteorology, eugenics, and psychometrics. Although he was by no means the first person to study fingerprints, he is generally acknowledged as being the first person to analyzc the subject in scientific detail, to offer a mathematical proof of the value of fingerprints in identifying specific individuals, and to outline the basic principles by which fingerprints can be used in forensic analysis. His first published work on the subject was an article published in the journal *Nature* in 1888, "Personal Identification and Description." He later wrote more than two dozen additional papers on the subject and three books, *Finger Prints* (1892), *Decipherment of Blurred Finger Prints* (1893), and *Fingerprint Directories* (1895).

Calvin H. Goddard, served in the U.S. Army, attaining the rank of colonel; was professor of police science at Northwestern University; and was military editor of the *Encyclopedia Britannica* and the *American Journal of Police Science.* Goddard was particularly interested in the study of ballistics and developed two devices—the comparison microscope and the helixometer—that enabled the comparison of bullets fired from two weapons. By examining characteristic markings on the bullet, Goddard was able to determine whether the two weapons used to fire the bullet were or were not one and the same. Goddard is credited with providing crucial evidence that helped solve the famous St. Valentine's Day massacre in Chicago in 1929. Goddard's successful work on this case led to the establishment of the nation's first crime laboratory at Northwestern University. While teaching at Northwestern, Goddard also offered the first courses in police science ever presented at an American college or university.

Henry Goddard, a member of London's first police force, the Bow Street Runners, and later the first chief constable of Northamptonshire, England. Goddard earned a reputation as a conscientious and efficient law enforcement officer who is probably best known today for his use of ballistic analysis in solving a London murder in 1835. Goddard compared certain characteristic marks on a bullet used in the crime with the mold from which it was made, providing an identification of the person who used the weapon in the crime.

Nehemiah Grew, an English botanist whose most famous work was *Anatomy of Plants*, published in 1682. Grew made some of the earliest studies of the surface of hands and feet and made detailed drawings of the ridges, furrows, and pores on the palms of hands and the soles of feet. His contributions have led to his designation as the father of dactyloscopy, the study of fingerprints and their comparison. He earned his medical degree at Leiden University in 1671 and maintained a very successful medical practice in London for many years, while continuing his research on plants. He was elected to the Royal Society in 1671 and later served as secretary of the society and editor of its *Philosophical Transactions*.

Hans Gross, from 1869 to 1897, an examining judge in the Austrian province of Styria. Gross is sometimes called the father of modern scientific criminology. He became a judge at the age of 22 at a time when persons holding that position were expected to perform a wide array of tasks that included crime investigator, prosecutor, and jurist. He was appalled at the low level of crime investigation and enforcement carried out within his jurisdiction and decided to encourage the use of any and all scientific methods to improve the quality of law enforcement within his province. In 1893, he published his classic work *Handbuch für Untersuchungsrichter* (later published in English as *Criminal Investigation*), which summarized his research and theories of scientific criminal investigation. The book was to go through six editions and was popular throughout the Western world. After leaving his post as judge in Styria, he served as professor of penal law at Czernowitz from 1897 to 1902, at Prague from 1902 to 1905, and finally at Graz, from 1905 until his death in 1915. In 1912, he founded the Institute of Criminalistics at Graz, from which his students carried his philosophy of the scientific investigation of crime throughout Europe. Gross also founded the journal *Kriminologie* and introduced the term *criminalistics* as a synonym for "forensic science."

Sir Edward Richard Henry, a member for 28 years of the Indian Civil Service posted at Fort William in Bengal. In 1891, Henry was appointed inspector general of the Bengal Police. A year later, the department adopted Alphonse Bertillon's system of anthropometry for the identification of criminals. Having read Francis Galton's essays on fingerprinting, however, Henry was also interested in pursuing the use of this technique as a system of identification. Between July 1896 and February 1897, Henry worked on a system by which fingerprints could be collected, filed, and searched in parallel with the anthropometric system also in use. Within a matter of months, it was obvious that a choice between the two systems should be made, and a royal commission appointed for that purpose unanimously recommended the use of fingerprinting rather than anthropometry. In 1901, he was recalled from his post in India and appointed assistant commissioner of Scotland Yard in charge of the Criminal Investigation Department. Later the same year, he established the first fingerprint bureau in the police agency, and in 1903, he was named commissioner of Scotland Yard, a post he held until 1918.

William James Herschel, a British civil servant who worked for the Indian Civil Service in the Hooghly district of Calcutta (now Kolkata). Herschel is widely credited with being one of the first persons in a position of authority to use fingerprints for the purpose of personal identification. He required native workers under his authority to affix their handprints to official documents to guarantee their authenticity. Some years later, a dispute arose as to who it was that should receive credit for inventing the use of fingerprinting for identification purposes. Some critics argue that Herschel used fingerprinting more for the purpose of frightening workers than for identification. Still, he was the first person to collect large numbers of prints that he saved for future reference over long periods of time.

Sir Alec Jeffreys, discoverer of the restriction fragment length polymorphism (RFLP) technique for the amplification of small segments of DNA. Along with the PCR (polymerase chain reaction) procedure invented by Kary Mullis in 1993, RFLP is one of the two widely used methods for increasing the length of DNA segments, permitting them to be analyzed and identified as belonging to some specific individual. Jeffreys majored in biochemistry at Merton College, Oxford University, and was awarded his Ph.D. in human genetics by Oxford in 1975. After completing his postdoctoral studies, Jeffreys accepted an appointment as lecturer in the Department of Genetics at the University of Leicester, where he has been employed ever since. Jeffreys has received a number of awards and honors in recognition of his work with RFLP, including the Colworth Medal for Biochemistry of the Biochemical Society (1985), the Linnean Bicentenary Medal for Zoology of the Linnean Society (1987), the Carter Medal of the Clinical Genetics Society (1987), the Davy Medal of the Royal Society (1987), the Allen Award of the American Society of Human Genetics (1992), the Gold Medal for Zoology of the Linnean Society of London (1994), and the Albert Einstein World of Science Award of the World

Cultural Council (1996). In 1994, Jeffreys was knighted by Queen Elizabeth II for his services to science and technology.

Thomas Jennings, the first person convicted in the United States on the basis of fingerprint evidence. On September 19, 1910, Clarence Hiller was found murdered in his home in Chicago, Illinois. In a matter of hours, Thomas Jennings, a convicted burglar, was found in the vicinity of the Hiller home and arrested for the murder. The strongest piece of evidence presented in the state's case against Hiller was a clean set of fingerprints left by the murderer on the newly painted walls of the Hiller home. Those prints matched prints taken from Jennings. The jury found the evidence compelling and convicted Jennings of the murder. Upon appeal, the trial court's decision was upheld on December 21, 1911, and Jennings was executed on February 16, 1912.

Leonarde Keeler, criminologist and important contributor to the development of the modern polygraph. Keller was born in North Berkeley, California, in 1903, and worked for the Berkeley Police Department during high school. At the time, John A. Larson was building one of the earliest models of the modern polygraph, a machine that was, however, awkward to work with. Keller made a number of improvements in the machine and, perhaps most important, decided to add a device for measuring the electrical conductivity of skin to blood pressure, pulse, and respiration rate already recorded by Larson's invention. Keeler's machine proved to be more efficient and easier to work with than Larson's model, and it was soon adopted by police departments across the nation. Keeler continued to make improvements in the polygraph for the rest of his life, during which he worked at Northwestern University's Scientific Crime Detection Laboratory (1930–38) and as a private polygraph consultant (1938–49). He died in Sturgeon Bay, Wisconsin, on September 20, 1949.

Alexandre Lacassagne, longtime professor of forensic medicine at the University of Lyon, France. Lacassagne was a leading figure in the development of a number of forensic techniques. For many years, he was an ardent supporter of anthropometry, and he carried out some of the first research on the information that can be adduced from blood spot patterns at the scene of a crime. He was also a pioneer in the study of ballistics, although he limited his analysis to only the most superficial markings produced on a bullet as the result of its being fired from a weapon. Lacassagne also had a strong influence on the development of forensic science in France and other parts of Europe through his teaching, lecturing, consulting, and training of students in criminalistics. In 1914, Lacassagne founded the Musée d'Histoire de la Médecine et de la Pharmacie (Museum of the History of Medicine and Pharmacy) in Lyon. He died as the result of an accident in 1924.

John Augustus Larson, Canadian-born physiologist often referred to as the father of polygraphy because of his early research on the design of polygraph machines. In 1921, August Vollmer, chief of police at Berkeley, California, asked Larson to develop a machine that would help determine when suspects were telling the truth during an interrogation and when they were lying. Larson constructed a machine that he first called a cardio-pneumo-psychograph, which measured pulse rate, respiratory rate, and blood pressure simultaneously. Larson later modified the name of the machine, calling it simply a lie detector. Vollmer and Larson tried out the machine first on the police chief himself and later on suspects in a number of crimes. They were delighted to find that it was generally able to distinguish between true statements and false statements. Larson also developed an interviewing technique called the R/I (for relevant/irrelevant) procedure, in which questions relevant to the case being investigated were intermixed with questions irrelevant to the case. Larson later became a forensic psychiatrist and worked at a number of hospitals, prisons, and other institutions.

Edmond Locard, a student of the renowned Alphonse Bertillon, assistant to the famous Alexandre Lacassagne, and founder of the Laboratoire de Police Scientifique in Lyon, France, in 1912. Locard earned his medical degree at the University of Lyon in 1902 and, eight years later, convinced the Lyon police department to provide him with two attic rooms and two assistants to establish a forensics laboratory. In his laboratory, Locard translated many of the theoretical ideas proposed by Hans Gross, Bertillon, and Lacassagne into actual methods and procedures that could be used in the analysis of crimes. He is perhaps best known today for his enunciation of the principle, Locard's Exchange Principle, that a criminal always leaves behind some piece of evidence at a crime scene. "Wherever he steps, whatever he touches, whatever he leaves, even unconsciously, will serve as a silent witness against him," Locard wrote. "Not only his fingerprints or his footprints, but his hair, the fibers from his clothes, the glass he breaks, the tool mark he leaves, the paint he scratches, the blood or semen he deposits or collects. All of these and more, bear mute witness against him." That principle is probably the single most fundamental guideline used by forensic scientists in their analysis of crime scenes. Locard also founded the Institute of Criminalistics in Lyon.

Cesare Lombroso, Italian criminologist who is best known for his theory that criminal tendencies are inherited and not a characteristic trait found to a greater or lesser degree in all humans. Lombroso believed that criminals constitute a specific type of humans with recognizable physical characteristics. Discovering those characteristics could then lead to a tool in the identification of recidivist criminals and a dramatic reduction in crime by preventing its occurrence. Trained as a physician, Lombroso served as professor of diseases of the mind at the University of Pavia and head of the insane asylum at Pesaro. He was also professor of medical law and psychiatry at the University of Turin. In the mid-1890s, Lombroso invented one of the first polygraphs, a device that measured blood pressure and pulse as an indication of a person's truthfulness. He called the machine a hydrosphygmograph. The addition of devices to measure respiratory rate and galvanic skin response resulted in the machine now known as a polygraph.

David Lykken, a member of the departments of psychology and psychiatry at the University of Minnesota for over 60 years. Lykken was interested in a wide variety of topics in the field of psychology, including behavioral genetics, psychopathology, psychophysiology, and lie detection. He is perhaps best remembered for his development of the guilty knowledge test (GKT), a protocol used in polygraph testing in which answers to some of the questions asked are known only to someone with knowledge of the crime. Lykken wrote extensively about the uses and abuses of polygraph testing, pointing out that the polygraph is not really a lie detector, but simply a way of measuring physiological responses to questions asked by the operator. The polygraph might or might not provide useful information in crime detection and other applications, he said, depending on a number of factors, including the questions asked and the interpretations possible from the responses given by the subject.

Herbert Leon MacDonell, director of the Laboratory of Forensic Science in Corning, New York, is an expert on many types of forensic analysis. He is the inventor of the MAGNA brush for lifting fingerprints from specialized types of materials, including tissue paper and human skin. The MAGNA brush is the only device available for collecting prints from the skin. He is also one of the world's foremost authorities on blood spatter patterns, the patterns produced when blood released during a violent crime creates distinctive formations on floors, walls, furniture, and other objects. MacDonnell has taught and lectured in many countries around the world and has served as an expert witness in a number of important civil and criminal trials, including those involving the trials of O. J. Simpson and Jean Harris and the murders of Robert Kennedy and Martin Luther King, Jr. He is the author of four books on blood stain pattern analysis. After having taught at Corning Community College and Elmira College, both in New York State, he founded the Bloodstain Evidence Institute in 1973.

Sir James Mackenzie, English physician who lived from 1853 to 1925 and invented a primitive form of the polygraph. Mackenzie specialized in cardiology and operated both a cardiac clinic and a cardiac ward in London, at which he studied a large number of heart disorders and trained young physicians in his special field of expertise. Mackenzie also invented a number of instruments for use in his research and clinical work, among them a device to measure arterial and venous pulse simultaneously. Although the device was originally developed to measure changes in heart rhythm associated with cardiac disorders, Mackenzie recognized its potential applications in determining when a person was telling the truth or not. The principle of his machine was later incorporated into the earliest polygraphs developed in the United States in the 1920s.

Marcello Malpighi, Italian anatomist of the 17th century. One of the most widely respected biologists of his time, Malpighi became an expert in the use of the newly invented microscope in the analysis of plant and animal materials. He studied the movement of blood through the capillaries and the structure of the lung, brain, spleen, liver, and kidneys. He conducted thorough anatomical studies of the chick, silkworm, and a variety of plants. In 1686, Malpighi became one of the first scholars to mention the existence of characteristic fingerprint patterns, although he made no mention of potential applications for this knowledge. He served as professor of anatomy at the University of Bologna from 1666 to 1691.

William Moulton Marston, credited with having invented the first modern polygraph in 1915 while still a graduate student at Harvard University. In addition to his work with lie detectors, Marston was a prominent psychologist and author of *Emotions of Normal People*, which became a classic in the field of DISC (dominance/inducement/steadiness/compliance) theory of behavioral science. Marston is also known for having created with his wife Elizabeth the comic strip character Wonder Woman.

Luke May, a private detective and consulting forensic scientist, sometimes known as "America's Sherlock Holmes." Essentially self-taught in the principles of forensic science, May was one of the first practitioners in the field to employ a wide variety of tools and techniques for the investigation of crimes. Well before the establishment of crime laboratories in municipal and state police departments, May created his own such research facility where he conducted his own investigations and conducted classes for police officers.

Robert Wilson McClaughry, warden of the U.S. penitentiary at Leavenworth, Kansas, from 1899 to 1913. A graduate of Monmouth College in Illinois, McClaughry was active in Republican politics for many years and with his brother founded and operated the "Carthage Republican" newspaper. He enlisted in the army at the beginning of the Civil War and was ultimately promoted to the rank of major. President Abraham Lincoln appointed him paymaster of the army in 1864. At the war's conclusion, he was involved in a number of business ventures until he was appointed warden of the Illinois State Prison in 1874. He later served as warden of the Pennsylvania State Reformatory, as superintendent of the Illinois

State Reformatory, as warden of the Illinois State Penitentiary, for a second time, and finally as warden at Leavenworth. McClaughry was long known as a vigorous advocate of the scientific approach to forensic science and in 1887 first introduced the use of bertillonage at the Illinois State Penitentiary. As warden at Leavenworth, he also introduced the use of fingerprinting as a means of identifying prisoners at the facility.

Robert Melias, the first person anywhere in the world to be convicted on the basis of DNA typing evidence. In November 1987, Melias broke into the home of a 45-year-old disabled woman, stole her jewelry, and raped her. In such circumstances, lawyers for the defense might reasonably be expected to suggest that the victim's identification of their client was based on mistaken identity, especially given the traumatic circumstances involved. In this case, however, law enforcement officials were able to collect samples of semen from the victim's petticoat, which they matched with DNA taken from a sample of blood given by Melias. The testing laboratory placed the likelihood of a match in this case at one in four million, a result that convinced Melias to change his plea from innocent to guilty. He was convicted of the crime and sentenced to eight years in prison for rape and five years for burglary.

Angelo Mosso, Italian physiologist who discovered that a person's breathing rate and blood flow to the brain changes when presented with certain stimuli. Mosso was trained as a physician and taught pharmacology and physiology at the University of Turin. He is perhaps best known for his studies of changes in blood flow to the brain following surgical procedures on the skull. He developed a variety of instruments to measure pulse rate and rate of breathing under a variety of conditions, such as sleep, emotional reactions, and mental activity. One of the instruments he invented, the sphygmomanometer, later became an essential part of the modern polygraph.

Kary Banks Mullis, inventor of the polymerase chain reaction (PCR) for the amplification of DNA segments, an accomplishment for which he was awarded the 1993 Nobel Prize in chemistry. Mullis attended the Georgia Institute of Technology and received his Ph.D. in biochemistry from the University of California at Berkeley in 1973. After completing his postdoctoral studies, he took a job at the Cetus Corporation in Berkeley, where he was assigned to work on oligonucleotides, organic molecules consisting of long chains of similar groups. Four years later, he conceived of a method by which very small strands of DNA can be amplified many times over to produce samples of a size that permits extensive analysis. Mullis's claims for the discovery of the PCR technique have been the subject of extensive criticism, and questions have been raised as to how credit for that accomplishment should (if at all) be shared with colleagues working in the field. In any case, the polymerase chain reaction has become an essential key in the forensic analysis of DNA samples. In recent years, Mullis has also been the source of some controversy because of his non-conventional views of topics such as AIDS (he does not believe it is caused by the HIV virus); global warming (he does not believe that human activities affect the Earth's average annual temperature); and destruction of the ozone layer (he does not believe that chlorofluorocarbons are responsible for the destruction of ozone in the stratosphere).

Peter Neufeld, professor at Fordham University School of Law, and cofounder with Barry Scheck of the Innocence Project, a program designed to assist wrongly convicted individuals in obtaining exoneration of the crimes for which they were convicted. Neufeld and Scheck became interested in DNA typing as a forensic tool and were defense lawyers in one of the most famous early cases involving DNA typing, *People v. Castro*, in 1988. While still at the Benjamin N. Cardozo School of Law at Yeshiva University, Neufeld and Scheck founded the Innocence Project, a program staffed primarily by law students at Cardozo operating under the supervision of faculty members. To date, the project has resulted in the exoneration of more than 200 wrongfully convicted men and women. Neufeld is coauthor with Scheck and Jim Dwyer of *Actual Innocence: Five Days to Execution, and Other Dispatches from the Wrongly Convicted*, a book that relates the stories of wrongfully convicted individuals. He is in wide demand as a speaker on the use of DNA typing for such cases.

Mathieu Orfila, a physician and professor of chemistry, often called the father of forensic toxicology. Born on the island of Minorca (Spain), Orfila studied medicine at the universities of Barcelona and Valencia. He traveled to Paris in 1807 to continue his medical studies and became a student of the famous French chemist Louis-Nicolas Vauquelin. After completing his studies with Vauquelin in 1811, Orfila became a private lecturer in chemistry and began work on the book for which he is best known, *Traité des poisons ou Toxicologie générale (*Treatise on poisons, or general toxicology*)*, published in 1813. He later wrote four more books dealing with toxicology, *Eléments de chimie médicale (Fundamentals of Medical Chemistry;* 1817), *Leçons de médecine legale* (Lessons in legal medicine; 1823), *Traité des exhumations juridiques* (Treatise on legal exhumation; 1830), and *Recherches sur l'empoisonnement par l'acide arsénieux* (Research on poisoning with arsenic acid; 1841).

James W. Osterburg, for many years chair of the Department of Criminal Justice at the University of Illinois at Chicago. In 1977, Osterburg suggested a method for determining the statistical probability of finding two fingerprints being exactly the same. He based his model on the frequency with which various minutiae in the prints are likely to be the same and the effect of empty spaces in the prints' occurring. Osterburg's model was published in the December 1977 issue of the *Journal of the American Sta-*

tistical Association. Osterburg was a highly respected criminologist who served as a consultant to the U.S. Department of State and the U.S. Department of Justice, as well as participating in the investigation and prosecution of thousands of criminal cases. He was the author of *Criminal Investigation: A Method for Reconstructing the Past.*

Jan Evangelista Purkinje, Austro-Hungarian physiologist and poet, credited for having discovered sweat pores and being the first researcher to make note of distinct fingerprint patterns, of which he identified nine distinct forms. Purkinje never commented on the possible use of fingerprint patterns as a means of personal identification, however. He is probably better known for a number of important contributions in the fields of physiology and histology. He was the first person, for example, to use a microtome rather than a razor blade to prepare very thin slices of tissue. Purkinje also made a number of breakthrough discoveries about the process of vision. He is also well known in his native land (now the Czech Republic) as a great poet and strong nationalist. He died on July 28, 1869, at the age of 82.

Lambert-Adolphe-Jacques Quételet (Adolphe Quételet), Belgian social statistician. Quételet was trained in mathematics and astronomy, but became more interested in the use of statistics to describe human characteristics and behavior. In 1835, he published his best known work, *A Treatise on Man, and the Development of His Faculties,* in which he explained how human physical and moral characteristics can be analyzed and categorized by the use of statistical techniques. In his 1871 book *Anthropometry, or the Measurement of Different Faculties in Man,* Quételet is credited with having laid down the fundamental principles of the science of anthropometry, in which certain physical characteristics are thought to be correlated with criminal tendencies. He called his method of analysis *social mechanics.*

Barry C. Scheck, professor of law and director of the Innocence Project at the Benjamin N. Cardozo School of Law, Yeshiva University. Scheck earned his B.S. at Yale University in 1971 and his J.D. at the University of California at Berkeley in 1974. Since 1978, he has been on the faculty at the Cardozo School of Law, where he specializes in criminal law and forensic DNA cases. In 1988, he and colleague Peter Neufeld founded the Innocence Project, a program whose mission is to exonerate individuals who have been convicted for crimes they did not commit. Evidence from DNA typing is used to achieve this objective and as of 2007, more than 200 wrongly convicted individuals have been released from prison as a result of the Innocence Project's efforts. Scheck also serves as a commissioner on the New York Forensic Science Review Board, a body that regulates all crime and forensic DNA laboratories in the state.

Thomas Taylor, a microscopist at the U.S. Department of Agriculture (USDA) during the last quarter of the 19th century. Little is known about

Taylor except for the fact that he was one of the first individuals in the United States to recognize the potential value of fingerprints as a means of identifying individuals. He expressed his ideas in popular and scholarly journals such as the *American Journal of Microscopy*, *Popular Science*, and *Scientific American*, although those ideas appeared to have had little or no impact on the law enforcement community. A report of a speech he gave in 1877 suggested that Taylor believed that palm prints and fingerprints could be used for the purpose of identification, especially in criminal cases.

Eugène-François Vidocq, founder and chief of the world's first detective force, the Sûreté of Paris in 1810. Vidocq's early life would seem to have qualified him for almost any career other than law enforcement. He was in trouble with the law almost constantly for the first 35 years of his life, as a burglar, murderer, smuggler, and privateer. In 1809, he offered his services to law enforcement officials of the French government in return for amnesty for his long record of crimes. The following year he was allowed to form France's (and the world's) first formal police force, consisting of a dozen detectives, most of whom, like Vidocq, gave up a life of crime to become law enforcement officers.

August Vollmer, longtime chief of police in Berkeley, California, and sometimes referred to as the father of modern law enforcement in the United States. When Vollmer arrived in Berkeley from his native New Orleans, Louisiana, in 1904, he was chosen town marshal after single-handedly preventing a potentially disastrous collision between a railroad freight car and passenger coach. In his new position, he became fascinated with the problems of law enforcement but found virtually nothing on the subject written in the United States. Instead, he collected and devoured a number of European publications on the subject, including Hans Gross's *Criminal Psychology* and Eugène-François Vidocq's *Memoirs*. Over time, Vollmer built a modern police force in Berkeley that became a model for law enforcement agencies throughout the nation. For example, he created a bicycle patrol, established the first system of centralized police records, developed a call box network, provided police patrol cars with radios, and required that all Berkeley police officers have a college degree and be trained in marksmanship. In 1907, Vollmer was elected president of the California Association of Police Chiefs in spite of the fact that Berkeley had not yet created that office. In 1916, he persuaded the University of California at Berkeley to offer courses in criminology, a step generally acknowledged as the beginning of academic programs in forensic science in the United States. Vollmer was also the first law enforcement official to make use of early lie detector devices in police investigations.

Juan Vucetich, criminologist and one-time director of the Center for Dactyloscopy (the study of fingerprints) in Buenos Aires, Argentina. Born in

Hvar, Dalmatia (now Croatia), in 1858, Vucetich emigrated to Argentina in 1882 and took a position in the La Plata Police Office of Identification and Statistics. He soon became interested in both anthropometry and fingerprint analysis, the latter after reading about Francis Galton's experiments on the subject. He began to collect fingerprints and to develop a logical system by which they could be classified and used for purposes of identification. In 1892, he was able to provide evidence that led to the conviction of a woman for the murder of her children, an accomplishment that earned him widespread recognition for his skills in fingerprint analysis. At the time, he decided to abandon the use of anthropometry in favor of fingerprint analysis, making Argentina the first nation in the world to do so. Vucetich's best known work was a general summary of his research, *Dactiloscopía Comparada*, published in 1904. In addition to his work in La Plata, he traveled widely collecting fingerprints from people in many parts of the world and lecturing and consulting on the use of fingerprints in forensic science. In his honor, a region of Buenos Aires has been named for Vucetich, as have the La Plata police academy (Escuela de policia Juan Vucetich) and the police Center for Forensics Examinations (Centar za kriminalistička vještačenja) in Zagreb, Croatia.

Charles E. Waite, a special investigator in the office of the New York Attorney General during the early decades of the 20th century. Waite is best known for his research that led to the first catalog containing manufacturing data on weapons and ammunition. He is reported to have test-fired every weapon made by the 12 most important weapons manufacturers in the world and then collected data from these firings into a single catalog available for the use of any law enforcement officer in the nation. Waite also collaborated with Dr. Max Poser of the Bausch & Lomb Optical Company in the development of the comparison microscope, a device that enables simultaneous examination of the markings on two bullets. In 1925, Waite joined with three other forensic experts, Calvin H. Goddard, Philip O. Gravelle, and John H. Fischer, to establish the Bureau of Forensic Ballistics in New York City.

CHAPTER 5

GLOSSARY

The terms used in discussions of forensic research, law enforcement, and DNA typing are drawn from a variety of fields, including science, technology, engineering, law, philosophy, religion, and business. This chapter provides definitions for some of the most common terms and phrases used in these fields.

abridged writing A shorthand method of describing human characteristics invented by Alphonse Bertillon in his system of anthropometry.

admissibility The property of being acceptable at a legal trial.

allele One of two or more alternative forms of a gene or genetic marker.

allelic ladder In DNA typing, a term that refers to a set of DNA fragments of precise and known size that can be used to estimate the size of an unknown DNA fragment.

amplification The process by which a single copy of DNA is reproduced many times over as a result of the polymerase chain reaction.

annealing The step during a polymerase chain reaction in which a DNA primer is attached to a segment of DNA to be reproduced.

anthropometry A system for identifying individuals based on body characteristics, such as size, breadth, and distance between certain anatomical parts.

antigen A foreign material present in the body capable of causing an adverse reaction, such as an allergic reaction (an allergen) or a disease.

arch A fingerprint pattern in which ridges enter on one side of the impression and flow out the other side with a wave in the center. Arches are classified as plain or tented depending on the details of their structure.

autorad *See* **autoradiograph.**

autoradiograph An X-ray photograph that shows marks produced radioactively or by means of chemiluminescence in the analysis of a DNA fragment.

ballistic fingerprint A set of unique markings left on a fired bullet and cartridge case by the weapon from which the bullet or cartridge case was fired.

Glossary

ballistics The science of the motion of projectiles. In forensics, three types of ballistics are of interest: interior ballistics, which deals with the properties of the projectile while still in a weapon; exterior ballistics, which involves the characteristics of the projectile as it travels through the air; and terminal ballistics, which is the study of the way a projectile penetrates a material.

base pair Either of the two nitrogen base combinations (guanine and cytosine or thymine and adenine) that is found in a DNA molecule.

bertillonage *See* **anthropometry.**

bifurcation A fingerprint characteristic; the point at which one friction ridge divides into two friction ridges.

blood alcohol concentration (BAC) The percentage of alcohol found in a person's blood.

brain wave fingerprinting A procedure (still experimental) that uses changes in brain wave activity to determine the veracity of that person's statements about an event when a person is presented with certain verbal and visual stimuli.

bridge A connecting friction ridge between and at generally right angles to parallel running ridges.

caliber The diameter of the bore of a rifled firearm, usually expressed in hundredths of an inch.

cardiograph The component of a polygraph test that records blood pressure, blood volume, and heart rate.

career criminal A term used to describe an individual who is arrested numerous times for participation in criminal acts.

characterization The process by which a sample of material is identified as belonging to some specific category.

chromatography A chemical procedure by which the components of a mixture are separated by being passed along a filter paper (paper chromatography), a stream of gas (gas chromatography), or some other material.

cold case A criminal case for which no resolution has been reached, although the case is still open for investigation.

cold hit An event in which DNA collected at the scene of a crime is matched against DNA from some individual whose DNA sample already resides in a DNA database.

Combined DNA Index System (CODIS) A database operated by the Federal Bureau of Investigation (FBI) that enables federal, state, and local crime labs to exchange and compare DNA profiles electronically.

comparison microscope A viewing device that consists of two microscopes joined by an optical bridge with a split screen that enables a viewer to see both fields at the same time.

confirmatory test A test that is performed to authenticate some association between two variables with a high degree of probability. See also **presumptive test.**

control question test The most commonly used test in polygraph testing in which certain questions for which the answer is known are asked.

crime gun database A database that contains ballistic fingerprints of firearms. The National Integrated Ballistic Information Network (NIBIN) Program of the Bureau of Alcohol, Tobacco, and Firearms (ATF) is an example of such a database.

criminalistics The analysis, comparison, identification, and interpretation of evidence collected in a crime.

criminology The study of crime and criminal behavior.

dactylography A term sometimes used to describe the analysis of fingerprints.

dactyloscopy *See* **dactylography.**

database An organized collection of information.

***Daubert* hearing** A court session held prior to a regular trial to determine which scientific evidence will be admissible in that trial.

denaturation The process by which the three-dimensional structure of a protein or nucleic acid molecule is destroyed by the addition of heat, chemicals, or some other agent. In DNA typing, the term refers specifically to the process by which a DNA molecule is uncoiled and/or separated into its two constituent strands.

deoxyribonucleic acid (DNA) A class of organic compounds found in the cells of almost all living organisms that directs protein synthesis and the transmission of genetic characteristics.

digital fingerprint A term sometimes used for traditional fingerprinting that uses prints from fingertips, the palm of the hand, and footprints, in contrast to **DNA fingerprinting.** *See also* **fingerprint.**

divergence A fingerprint pattern that consists of the separation of two friction ridges that have been running parallel or nearly parallel.

DNA databank A collection of DNA records, obtained from local, state, and/or federal sources, of individuals who have been convicted of a crime. *See also* **Combined DNA Index System.**

DNA fingerprinting *See* **DNA typing.**

DNA primer *See* **DNA probe.**

DNA probe A synthetically produced DNA fragment designed to match some specific DNA target. Also known as a DNA primer.

DNA profiling *See* **DNA typing.**

DNA typing A process by which fragments of DNA are used to identify the person or other organism from which they came.

DRUGFIRE A now obsolete system for comparing ballistic fingerprints developed by the Federal Bureau of Investigation (FBI), and since replaced by the Integrated Ballistic Identification System (IBIS) operated by the Bureau of Alcohol, Tobacco, and Firearms (ATF).

Glossary

electrodermal response (EDR) A measure of the electrical conductivity of skin in a polygraph test, reflecting the subject's physiological response to a question asked by the examiner.

electrophoresis A chemical test in which the components of a mixture are separated from each other on the basis of their differential rate of movement in an electric field.

ergonomics The study of the relationship between the human body and the working environment.

event-specific polygraph A polygraph test that is carried out in relationship to some specific incident, in which there is reasonable cause to believe that the person being examined may be involved in the case.

evidence Documents, records, testimony, material objects, or other things presented at a trial to prove the existence or nonexistence of a fact.

exon The section of a DNA or RNA molecule that carries instructions for making a protein.

exploratory test A general test of an individual, as in a polygraph examination, that deals with a broad range of issues.

extension The step during a polymerase chain reaction in which DNA polymerase enzymes add nucleotides to a segment of DNA specifically marked off by DNA primers.

false negative A result that indicates the absence of some condition that is, in fact, actually present.

false positive A result that indicates the presence of some condition that is, in fact, not actually present.

fingerprint The impression, visible or not, left when a person's finger(s) come into contact with a surface, leaving behind a characteristic pattern of ridges, grooves, whorls, arches, and other features by which the print can be identified. *See also* **latent fingerprint.**

forensic science The application of principles and technology from physics, chemistry, biology, and other sciences to the investigation of criminal activity and legal procedures related to such activity.

friction ridge *See* **ridge.**

galvanic skin response (GSR) A change in the electrical conductivity of skin that occurs in response to stress, anxiety, or some other emotional response. GSR is presumed by polygraph operators to indicate that a person is not telling the truth about a question asked during an examination.

gas chromatography *See* **chromatography.**

genetic fingerprinting *See* **DNA typing.**

grooves In digital fingerprinting: Valley-like regions of a fingerprint or a ballistic marking. In ballistic fingerprinting: Milled-out areas on the inside surface of a weapon's barrel or comparable markings produced on a bullet fired through a gun barrel.

hydrosphygmograph A primitive type of lie detector consisting of a water-filled jar with a rubber membrane covering its opening.

identification The determination of the chemical and physical properties of a substance with as much certainty as permitted by the tools and technology available.

inconclusive result A result obtained in any type of forensic test (such as DNA typing or polygraph testing) that is insufficient to determine the guilt or innocence of the person being examined.

individualization The concept that any individual piece of evidence of whatever kind can be conclusively linked to a specific individual.

infrared spectroscopy An analytical technique in which light produced by a heated object is divided into its component parts in order to determine the elements present in the object.

Integrated Ballistic Identification System (IBIS) An automated and computerized system for storing and classifying ballistic fingerprints made by a large range of weapons. IBIS is operated by the Bureau of Alcohol, Tobacco, and Firearms (ATF) of the U.S. Department of the Treasury.

in-test phase That portion of a polygraph test during which physiological data, such as galvanic skin response (GSR), heart rate, and blood pressure, are recorded in response to an examiner's questions.

intron A portion of a DNA molecule that does not code for the synthesis of a protein.

irrelevant question *See* **neutral question.**

islands Sections of a fingerprint in which ridges close in upon themselves.

junk DNA *See* **intron.**

latent fingerprint A fingerprint that is not visible to the naked eye, but which can be treated so as to make it visible.

lie detector Any device used to determine the veracity of a person's statements. The most common lie detector used today is the polygraph.

locus The position of a gene on a chromosome.

loops Closed segments in a fingerprint. Loops are classified as radial or ulnar, depending on the details of their structure.

luminescence The emission of visible light by a material when it is exposed to some form of radiation, such as infrared radiation.

mass spectrometer A device for determining the components of a compound or mixture on the basis of the movement of those components as they pass through a magnetic field.

minutiae Ridges, grooves, and other fingerprint details that are used to make identifications of the fingerprint.

morphological vocabulary A term used by Alphonse Bertillon to describe all of the exact language used to describe characteristic features of the human body.

multiplexing The process in the polymerase chain reaction (PCR) by which more than one locus on a DNA molecule is analyzed at the same time.

National Integrated Ballistic Information Network (NIBIN) A program established by the Bureau of Alcohol, Tobacco, and Firearms (ATF) in 1997 to make information available on ballistic fingerprints in federal, state, and local databases for use by all users of the network.

neutral question A question asked during a polygraph examination that is unrelated to the issue actually of interest in the test. *See also* **relevant question.**

ninhydrin A chemical used to detect fingerprints because it reacts with proteins present in the prints.

nucleotide A chemical compound consisting of the sugar deoxyribose, a phosphate group, and one of four nitrogen bases; the basic unit of a DNA molecule.

ordeal A test used to determine the veracity of a person's statements. More commonly used in primitive societies and involving the conduct of some act that is used to differentiate between truth-tellers and liars.

penology The study of prisons, prisoners, and the treatment of crime.

pH A measure of the acidity of an aqueous (water) solution, defined as the negative logarithm of the concentration of the hydrogen ion concentration.

physical evidence Any object or material that can be used to link a crime with a victim or a crime with a perpetrator or that can be used to prove that a crime has been committed.

plethysmograph An instrument used to measure changes in the size of an organ or some other part of the body as a result of changes in the amount of blood it contains.

pneumograph A device that records thoracic and/or abdominal breathing patterns.

polygraph An instrument consisting of a number of parts that record respiration rate, cardiovascular activity, and galvanic skin response (GSR) of the person being examined.

polymerase chain reaction (PCR) A method of DNA typing or DNA fingerprinting in which short segments of DNA are amplified and then analyzed and compared with standard references.

polymorphic Existing in more than one form, as in the various alleles that a gene may possess.

power of discrimination The ability of a test to distinguish between any two individuals, conditions, circumstances, or events chosen at random.

presumptive test A test that is performed when there is some reasonable basis for believing that some positive result will be obtained. *See also* **confirmatory test.**

profiling A procedure by which a particular individual is judged on the basis of certain characteristics that person shares with a larger group. Some characteristics used for profiling include skin color, type of clothing, language, and characteristic behaviors.

recidivism The tendency of a person to relapse into criminal behavior that he or she has exhibited in the past. Habitual or repeat criminals are recidivists.

relevant question A question asked during a polygraph test that has relevance to the issue being investigated in the examination. *See also* **neutral question.**

reliable A result is said to be reliable if it is repeated a number of times in response to the same question or stimulus. A reliable result need not be a valid (correct) result.

restriction enzymes Enzymes that "recognize" characteristic patterns of nucleotide sequences in DNA and that cut the DNA at specific points in that sequence.

restriction fragment length polymorphism (RFLP) A system for testing DNA samples to determine the individual from whom they have come.

ridge characteristics Patterns on a person's fingers, palms, or feet, such as arches and whorls, that can be used to identify a fingerprint as belonging to a specific individual.

ridges The raised markings on a person's fingers, palms, or feet partially responsible for the formation of fingerprints.

rifling The process by which spiral grooves are etched into the inner surface of a gun barrel.

short tandem repeats (STRs) Any tandem repeat with a relatively small number of repeating base pairs. *See also* **tandem repeat.**

sphygmomanometer An instrument used to measure blood pressure.

tandem repeat Any section of a DNA molecule in which a particular pattern of base pairs appears more than once.

valid A true or correct result.

whorl One of the three basic fingerprint patterns (along with arch and loop) in which ridges form at least one complete circuit. Whorls are classified as accidental, plain, double loop, or central pocket loop depending on the detail of their structures.

PART II

GUIDE TO FURTHER RESEARCH

CHAPTER 6

How to Conduct Research on Forensic Science and DNA Typing

Fingerprinting, ballistic testing, polygraphs, and DNA testing are subjects of interest to many people. This chapter suggests a number of ways in which researchers can learn more about the history, scientific background, and legal status of these forensic procedures. It provides suggestions about the use of print and electronic resources generally available to researchers. In addition, suggestions are offered for the somewhat specialized area of legal topics relating to fingerprinting, ballistic testing, polygraphs, and DNA typing.

PRINT SOURCES

For many centuries, the primary source of information on any topic has been the library. Libraries are usually buildings that hold materials known as *bibliographic resources*, books, magazines, newspapers, and other periodicals and documents, as well as audiovisual materials and other sources of information. General libraries tend to vary in size from small local facilities with only a few thousand books and periodicals to mammoth collections such as the Library of Congress in Washington, D.C.; the Bibliothèque Nationale de France, in Paris; and the British Library, in London, each of which holds millions of individual items. A list of the world's major general national libraries is online at "National Libraries of the World," http://www.ifla.org/VI/2/p2/nationallibraries.htm

Some libraries specialize in specific topics, ranging from business and education to medical research and the health sciences. Examples of specialized libraries are the Monroe C. Gutman Library (education) at Harvard University; the Gulf Coast Environmental Library in Beaumont, Texas; the

Jonsson Library of Government Documents at Stanford University; the Cornell Law Library, in Ithaca, New York; and the health sciences libraries maintained by many universities.

Specialized libraries often have information on a topic that is not available at most general libraries. At one time, that fact was not very helpful to someone who would have to travel to Berkeley, Princeton, or some other distant location to obtain the information he or she needed. Today most libraries, both general and specialized, have online catalogs that are entirely or partially available to anyone with access to a computer. These online catalogs often allow a researcher to locate a needed item, an item that can then be ordered through a local library by means of interlibrary loan. Further information about general and specialized libraries and about the use of interlibrary loan services can be obtained from your local school or community librarian. Law libraries affiliated with local, state, and federal governments and with law schools are often a good source of information on forensic issues, such as fingerprinting and DNA typing. A list of all law libraries in the United States and Canada can be found in *AALL Directory and Handbook*, published annually by the American Association of Law Libraries (AALL) and available at all AALL members or at the association's web site (http://www.aallnet.org/products/pub_handbook.asp).

Library Catalogs

The key to accessing the vast resources of any library is the card catalog. At one time, a card catalog consisted exclusively of a collection of cards stored in wooden cabinets and arranged by title, author, and subject of all the books and other materials owned by a library. Today, most libraries also have an electronic card catalog in which that information exists in electronic files that can be accessed through computers. Some libraries have eliminated the older, physical form of their card catalog, making it possible to access their collections only through the electronic card catalog. The electronic card catalog has the advantage of being available to researchers from virtually any location, compared to the traditional physical card catalog, which can be accessed only at the library itself.

Whether one searches a library's resources by means of its physical card catalog or its electronic equivalent, that search may take any one of a number of forms. One may, for example, search for the title of a publication, by the author, by subject matter, by certain key words, by publication date, or by some other criterion. While physical catalogs tend to use only the first three of these criteria, electronic catalogs often provide researchers with a wider range of options, options that can be explored by means of *advanced searches*. Advanced searches allow one to search for various combinations of words and numbers, combining some terms, and requiring that others be ignored. For example, one may wish to locate books that have been written on the subject of digital fingerprinting only between the years 2000 and 2005, only in English, and only by an author with the last name of Black. An advanced search allows these conditions to be used in looking for items in a catalog.

Advanced searches are very helpful when an initial search produces too many results. If one looks only for the subject *fingerprinting* in a catalog, for example, one may find hundreds or thousands of entries. For example, a search for that term in the online Summit search engine, which is used by all academic libraries in the state of Oregon, returns a total of 304 items. While not impossible, examining all the titles in that list would be time-consuming, especially if one knows in advance that he or she is interested in only one aspect of the subject. For example, if the topic of interest were really legal issues involving fingerprinting, an advanced search should be used that combined these terms, in the form "fingerprinting" and "law," "fingerprinting" and "legal issues," or some similar choice of search terms. Combinations such as these return only 45 items and one item, respectively, in the Summit system, far more manageable lists.

One of the key tools used in advanced searches is the Boolean operator. A Boolean operator is a term that tells a computer how it should treat the terms surrounding the term. The three most common Boolean operators are AND, OR, and NOT. If a computer sees two words or phrases connected by an AND, it understands that it should look only for materials in which *both* words or phrases occur. If the computer sees two words connected by an OR, it knows that it should search for any document that contains one word or phrase *or* the other, but not necessarily both. If the computer encounters two words or phrases connected by a NOT, it understands that it should ignore the specific category that *follows* the NOT when searching for the general category that precedes the NOT.

An important skill in searching for materials in either a library or on the Internet is to remember that documents are not always identified by a computer in the same terms in which a researcher is thinking of them. For example, a researcher may be interested in tracking down all books in a library on the subject of *DNA typing*. If he or she types that term into the library's catalog, a few hundred or a few thousand items may show up. What the researcher may not know is that many more items of interest may exist in the library's holdings. Other authors and/or librarians may use other terms to describe the same idea as expressed by *DNA testing*, *DNA fingerprinting*, *genetic fingerprinting*, *DNA profiling*, or some other term. Some terms that might also refer to articles or books on *DNA typing* are *forensic DNA*, *forensic medicine*, and *applications of DNA*. These terms do not mean exactly the same thing as *DNA typing*, but they are close enough to serve as search terms. But even these terms do not exhaust the possible range of identifiers that will produce materials of value to the researcher. Some of the other words and phrases that one might try include the following:

- RFLP (or restriction fragment length polymorphisms)
- PCR (or polymerase chain reaction)
- applications of DNA
- DNA analysis
- forensic genetics
- expert evidence (or evidence, expert)
- evidence, legal

The same approach is necessary, of course, in searching for more specialized areas of forensic science procedures. In looking for materials on the history of such procedures, one should search not only under fingerprinting, polygraphs, or DNA typing, but also under a variety of other variations, such as:

- forensic science—history
- history of fingerprinting
- chronology of lie detectors
- development of DNA fingerprinting

and so on.

One of the keys to success in finding all or most of the materials in a library on some given topic is to imagine as many different words and phrases as possible by which that topic might be identified.

SCHOLARLY ARTICLES

One area in which libraries continue to have an important advantage over Internet searching is in the use of scholarly articles. Anyone interested in forensic procedures such as fingerprinting, lie detection, and DNA typing issues will want to examine articles published in all kinds of periodicals, ranging from general interest newspapers, such as the *New York Times* and the *Washington Post*, to more specialized journals, such as the *Journal of Forensic Science*, *Journal of Forensic Identification*, *Science & Justice*, *FBI Law Enforcement Bulletin*, *Forensic Science Communications*, and *Forensic Science International*. Many libraries—especially academic and specialized libraries—subscribe to a wide variety of periodicals such as these, both general and specialized in character. Anyone who visits the library has access to these periodicals free of charge.

Those periodicals are, in almost all cases, also available online. Periodicals differ in their policies on accessing past articles. In some cases, they allow access free of charge to all articles to all users of the Internet. In other cases, they make some articles available at no cost, while a charge is assessed for accessing other articles. In the majority of cases, scholarly journals restrict access to articles to members of some particular professional society (such as the Forensic Science Society) and to readers who are willing to pay for an article. Non-members may purchase the right to read an article for a fee, which varies from periodical to periodical. In many cases, the fee is substantial, ranging from $10 to $35 per article. The general researcher will seldom be able to afford the purchase of every article found on the Internet on restricted sites. His or her choice, then, is to try locating that article in a local library (usually an academic library), requesting a copy of the article through interlibrary loan, or purchasing the article online from the journal publisher.

INTERNET SOURCES

Today, the resources of libraries have been greatly enhanced by the Internet, and its cousin, the World Wide Web. The Internet is a vast collection of networks, each containing very large amounts of information, generally accessible to almost any kind of individual computer. The Internet was first created for use by the U.S. military in 1969 and has since expanded to include networks of every imaginable kind from every part of the world.

WEB SITES

On the Internet, data are stored in web sites, locations where information about some specific topic is to be found. That information may range from the very specific to the very general. In the case of the forensic sciences, for example, one can find web sites that focus on topics as specific as a particular research study on DNA typing (such as "DNA Fingerprinting for Forensic Identification: Potential Effects on Data Interpretation of Subpopulation Heterogeneity and Band Number Variability" at http://www.ncbi.nlm.nih.gov/entrez/query.fcgi?cmd=Retrieve&db=PubMed&list_uids=2301401&dopt=Abstract) or as general as the overall subject of DNA typing research itself (such as "DNA Typing and Identification" at http://faculty.ncwc.edu/TOConnor/425/425lect15.htm).

A good place to begin in researching forensic technologies is with web sites whose primary or exclusive focus is on these subjects, web sites such as the following:

- "DNA Fingerprinting." URL: http://www.bergen.org/AAST/Projects/Gel/fingprint1.htm.

- "How Does Genetic Fingerprinting Work?" http://www.thenakedscientists.com/HTML/Columnists/dalyacolumn8.htm.
- "How Lie Detectors Work." http://people.howstuffworks.com/liedetector.htm.
- "Polygraph (Lie Detector)." http://skepdic.com/polygrap.html.
- "Fingerprint Patterns." http://www.policensw.com/info/fingerprints/finger07.html.
- "Fingerprinting." http://bennettkids.homestead.com/fingerprinting.html.
- "Ballistics." http://medlib.med.utah.edu/WebPath/TUTORIAL/GUNS/GUNBLST.html.
- "All about Ballistics in Solving Crime." http://www.crimelibrary.com/criminal_mind/forensics/ballistics/1.html.

One benefit of general purpose web sites of this kind is that they often provide links (connections) to other web sites with information on similar or related topics. The "How Stuff Works" web site listed above, for example, provides links to other How Stuff Works pages as well as to external web sites such as an article "Polygraph Results Often in Question," American Polygraph Association, American Association of Police Polygraphists, a web site AntiPolygraph.org, and a position statement by the Federation of American Scientists on polygraph policy.

Searching through web sites on the Internet involves three fundamental problems of which the researcher should always be aware: complexity, accuracy, and evanescence (instability). Internet web sites are related to each other in a complex, web-like fashion (hence the name World Wide *Web*), and not in a linear fashion, like the chapters in a book. When one goes looking through the Internet ("surfing the net"), one quickly heads off in dozens of different directions, often crossing and crisscrossing pathways and web sites. It is easy to get lost and forget how one arrived at a particular web site or how to get back to the beginning of a search string. One technique for keeping track of data is to print out every page that may seem to have some significance to one's research. That information may later prove to be of little or no value. But if it does turn out to be important, the researcher does not have to worry about finding it again at some time in the future. One can also mark the page containing the information as a "Favorite," using the toolbar in the web browser's menu, allowing one to return to that page if and when it is needed at a later time.

The second inherent problem with the Internet is the accuracy of web sites. Anyone can create his or her own web site with any kind of information at all on it. The information does not have to be true or accurate, and no outside monitor exists to tell a researcher whether the information is reliable or not. In searching for information on polygraph testing, for example, one web site could report that polygraph results are always correct and accepted by every court in the United States. Without outside references, there is no way of knowing which of these statements is (or are) actually factual. As a result, researchers must constantly be even more careful than they are with print materials (which are, at least, usually edited and fact checked) as to the accuracy of information found on the Internet. They can, for example, check other web sites or print materials on the same topic to verify that information given as facts is really true. They can also look carefully at web sites themselves to see if they appear to have some special argument about the forensic technology in question in their presentation.

Bias, and the inaccuracies it may include, is especially likely to occur in web sites on that deal with controversial issues. When people feel very strongly about a topic, they may accidentally or intentionally provide information that is incomplete, slanted, or simply wrong. Researching a topic such as polygraph testing, for example, requires a degree of caution and a willingness to double-check information more often than when conducting other forms of research.

The third problem in conducting online research is evanescence, or the tendency of web sites to disappear over time. Nothing is likely to be as frustrating for a researcher as to find a reference to a web site with what looks to be just the right information, only to receive the message "Web site not found." The web site has, usually for unknown reasons, been deleted, and is no longer available on the Internet.

However, it may not really be gone forever. Sometimes the web site's address has simply been changed, a possibility that the search engine may suggest by providing possible alternative leads to the site. Or, the web site may have been *cached*, that is, set aside in a "hidden" location in the computer's memory. The web site may then be accessed by asking the search engine to retrieve the desired page from its "hidden memory." Many "dead sites" have been stored on the Internet Archive (http://www.archive.org). A word of caution: Not every site is stored here, and users need to know the exact URL to access a site. Also, most sites archived have been stripped of all their image files.

SEARCH ENGINES

Probably the most important single tool one can use in searching the Internet is a search engine. Search engines are systems by which one can sift through the millions of web sites available online in order to find those that may contain information on some topic of interest. Search engines are amazing technological tools that accomplish this objective in a fraction of a second and then present the researcher with the names of web sites that are likely to be of interest.

Some of the most popular search engines now available include Google, Yahoo!, Dogpile, Ask, AllTheWeb, HotBot, Teoma, and LookSmart. (For an exhaustive review of search engines and related topics, see SearchEngine-Watch at http://searchenginewatch.com or SearchEngineJournal at http://www.searchenginejournal.com.) By far the most widely used of these engines is Google, which claims to search out more than 25 billion web sites.

Learning to use a search engine is similar to learning other skills: The longer one does the skill, the more one learns about the process and the better one becomes at it. The easiest approach is simply to type in a word or phrase in which one is interested and press "Enter." The problem is that "easy" in searching is often not "efficient." A search engine is likely to return the names of many web sites that have little or nothing to do with the topic of interest. For example, asking a search engine to look for *DNA fingerprinting* may produce a number of web sites that discuss books about DNA typing research, companies engaged in DNA typing research or the manufacture of equipment and materials for DNA typing, blogs (online personal journals) about DNA typing, or some other topic related to DNA typing research. While these topics may be of interest to a researcher, they may also be too specialized or too far afield from the researcher's main field of interest in DNA typing.

One way to avoid having too many unrelated web sites appear during a search is to be as specific as possible. If one wished to obtain information on the legal status of restriction fragment length polymorphisms testing (RFLP; a type of DNA fingerprinting) in the United States, for example, it would not be very efficient to start searching just for *DNA typing*. Even though that search probably would turn up web sites that discuss the question in which the researcher is interested, it would also produce many pages that have nothing to do with that specific topic. Instead, it would be more efficient to ask for more specific terminology, such as *restriction fragment length polymorphisms*, *RFLP*, or *legal status of DNA typing*, for example. An even more efficient approach is to ask for the specific topic in which one is interested, such as "legal status of restriction fragment length polymorphisms testing in the United States." Notice that words within quotation marks will be treated by the search engine as unitary terms.

This direct approach to searching has some inherent drawbacks. For example, a web site might use the phrase "restriction fragment length polymorphism" (leaving off the "s") and not recognize the precise search term entered by the researcher. Also, any web site where the term *polymorphism* (or any other word) is misspelled will not recognize the search term. Still, entering the exact phrase in which one is interested is a good start. If enough responses are not retrieved, one can make changes in the phrase.

For example, "legal status of restriction fragment length polymorphisms testing in the United States" can be re-entered as two or more phrases, such as "legal status," "restriction fragment length polymorphisms testing," "United States," or slight alterations can be made in the search phrase, such as "legal status of RFLP testing in the United States" or "legal status of restriction fragment length polymorphisms in the United States."

Trial-and-error and "practice, practice, practice" are two good ways to improve one's skills on Internet searching. Formal instruction is often very helpful also. One can learn a great deal from a brother or sister, a teacher, or a friend who has experience using the Internet. Instruction is also available on the Internet itself. For example, three web sites that provide tutorials on Internet searching are Learn the Net at http://www.learnthenet.com/english/index.html, Silwood Cyber Centre at http://www.silwoodonline.org.uk/cybercentre/learning.htm, and the University of California—Berkeley Internet Tutorial at http://www.lib.berkeley.edu/TeachingLib/Guides/Internet/FindInfo.html.

Another type of search engine that is often of value is the metasearch program. Metasearch engines (also known as *metacrawlers*) hunt through other search engines, collecting web sites in each of those search engines they believe to be the best matches of a researcher's search terms. Among the most popular metasearch engines now available are Dogpile, Vivisimo, Kartoo, Mamma, and SurfWax.

FORENSIC SCIENCE RESEARCH WEB SITES

Some of the most useful information about forensic science technologies is to be found in web sites that are wholly devoted to that subject. Those web sites may range in size from a single page to one with dozens or even hundreds of pages. The goals of such sites also range from providing a brief, general overview of the subject to covering as many aspects of the issue, such as scientific, technical, economic, social, and political as possible. An example of a general information web site is the one maintained by the American Polygraph Association, "Frequently Asked Questions," at http://www.polygraph.org/faq.cfm.

Controversies still remain about the use of some forensic technologies. The level of controversy varies from technology to technology. DNA typing, for example, is now widely accepted as a reliable and valid method of identifying an individual or a sample of living material. Digital fingerprinting has traditionally been widely accepted also, although questions have been raised in the past few years as to the scientific basis on which legal certainty has been based. And the forensic value of ballistic analysis and polygraph testing is still a subject of considerable debate both within the professional community of forensic scientists and among the general public.

These controversies are often an obvious or hidden part of web sites dealing with a forensic technology. For example, the American Polygraph Association web site mentioned above is operated by a professional organization consisting of individuals who make their living in the polygraph industry and so obviously believe in the validity of polygraph testing. Although it is unlikely that the web site contains inaccurate information, it would not be surprising for it to have some bias toward the use of polygraph testing. Many web sites make very clear their bias in one direction or another about a forensic technology. The web site AntiPolygraph.org (http://antipolygraph.org/) makes no secret of its views on polygraph testing. Its primary publication, for example, is entitled "The Lie Behind the Lie Detector."

Other web sites are more subtle about their own position on some forensic technology or another. Such web sites require that researchers note very carefully the sponsoring organization and look for indications that information provided may be biased in one direction or another.

LEGAL RESEARCH

Legal issues are, of course, a fundamental part of any discussion of forensic technologies, such as digital fingerprinting or ballistic analysis. The point of such technologies is to collect and analyze evidence that can be presented in a court of law so that judges and juries can make decisions about the guilt or innocence of individuals accused of a crime. So research on forensic technologies inherently requires that one become familiar with both library and Internet sources that contain information about federal, state, and local laws, regulations, and administrative rulings, and about court cases relating to the use of various forensic technologies.

FINDING LAWS AND REGULATIONS

The best places to begin a search for laws and regulations on any topic, including forensic technologies, are web sites that specialize in such information. The most dependable of these web sites are those maintained by a governmental agency or by some other organization (often a university) hired by a government agency to manage the web site. Some web sites with which every researcher should become familiar are the following:

- "U.S. Code Collection." http://www4.law.cornell.edu/uscode/. This web site is operated by Cornell University Law School and contains the complete text of the United States Code, the document in which all federal laws are to be found. Each of the 50 chapters of the code is collected into its own file and is searchable either by chapter or globally. The

U.S. Code is the first place to search for any law dealing with any type of forensic technology. The U.S. Code is also accessible by way of the Government Printing Office's web site, "GPOAccess," at http://www.gpoaccess.gov/uscode/index.html

- "FindLaw." http://lp.findlaw.com/. FindLaw is a web site intended for legal professionals, but it is accessible to laypersons also. The site has access to virtually every type of document in which either the professional or layperson might be interested, including federal, international, and state laws; court decisions at most levels and in most jurisdictions; resources by specific areas of practice (such as criminal law and military law); information on legal careers and legal resources; and specific information and resources for the legal community.
- USA.gov. http://www.usa.gov/. USA.gov is administered by the U.S. General Services Administration's Office of Citizen Services and Communications and is the first stop for any researcher wanting to know almost anything about the federal government. It is far more comprehensive than either the U.S. Code or FindLaw, which is both an advantage, in that it gives a broader view of many topics, and a disadvantage, in that it usually provides more information than one needs on a specific topic.
- "FedLaw." http://www.thecre.com/fedlaw/default.htm. FedLaw is a comprehensive source of information on federal laws and regulations. It was developed by Janice K. Kendenhall, who served for many years in the Federal Technology Service of the General Services Administration in Atlanta, Georgia. Although there is some overlap with other web sites, FedLaw tends to contain a broader range of topics, including federal laws, rules, and regulations; federal judicial decisions; some state laws; arbitration and mediation decisions; general research and reference sources; professional associations; and references to legal issues.
- "Thomas." http://thomas.loc.gov/. Thomas (named for Thomas Jefferson) is operated by the Library of Congress. It is the ultimate source of information on all legislative issues and contains the complete legislative history and text of all bills and resolutions introduced in the House and Senate, other activities in Congress, the *Congressional Record*, schedules and calendars of the two houses and their committees, information on all legislative committees, presidential nominations, treaties, and other government resources
- "LawGuru.com." http://www.lawguru.com/index.php. LawGuru.com is a privately owned web site operated by a California corporation that provides legal information for the legal profession, the general public, and students. Its law library contains a collection of federal and state laws,

laws of other nations, international treaties, legal directories, and a listing of law schools and libraries.

"Federal Government Resources—Laws and Regulations." http://www.lib.umich.edu/govdocs/fedlaws.html. Operated by the University of Michigan Documents Center, this web site contains documents on an extensive array of topics, including compilations such as the Code of Federal Regulations, Federal Register, Public Laws, United States Code; documents on individual topics such as abortion, copyright, crime, cyberspace, military justice, and regulations; and related topics, such as administrative law, presidential executive orders, Supreme Court decisions, municipal codes, state laws, international organization charters, treaties, and foreign laws.

FINDING COURT DECISIONS

Many of the web sites listed above provide access to court decisions at the federal, state, district, appeals, or other level. FindLaw is one of the most complete and easily accessible of those sources. Finding court decisions and understanding the terminology and abbreviations used in citations and decisions is sometimes difficult. For researchers with little background in legal matters, an excellent tutorial is available on the Internet. The tutorial is called Legal Research FAQ [frequently asked questions] and was authored by attorney Mark Eckenwiler in 1996. The tutorial provides a very readable and detailed explanation of the way court decisions are identified and how they can be located online and in print resources. The tutorial can be accessed by a number of pathways, one of which is http://www.faqs.org/faqs/law/research/part1/. A number of other web sites provide suggestions for searches in specific libraries or other sources. For example, Nolo Press sponsors an excellent web site called "Help with Legal Research" (http://www.nolo.com/statute/index.cfm) that answers almost every question the average researcher will have. An excellent overview on using the Internet for all kinds of legal research has also been made available by Lyonette Louis-Jacques, librarian and lecturer in law at University of Chicago Law School. That overview, "Legal Research Using the Internet," is available online at http://www.lib.uchicago.edu/~llou/mpoctalk.html.

CHAPTER 7

ANNOTATED BIBLIOGRAPHY

The bibliography of forensic technologies consists of a very large collection of books, articles, reports, brochures, pamphlets, Internet sites, and other resources. This chapter lists some of the most important of these resources. They are arranged in two ways, first by category: fingerprinting, ballistic analysis, anthropometry, polygraph testing, and DNA typing. Within each of these categories, resources are further subdivided according to type: books, articles, and Internet sites. Some overlap among categories occurs when a particular item can be listed under more than one kind of technology or more than one format (such as articles that are also available on the Internet).

GENERAL

BOOKS

Almirall, Jose R., and Kenneth G. Furton. *Forensic Science Explained: Guide for Understanding the Use of Science in the Administration of Justice*. Boca Raton, Fla.: CRC Press, 2005. This book is written primarily to explain the basic principles of forensic science to judges and juries, although it may be of interest also to members of the general public.

Bell, Suzanne. *The Facts On File Dictionary of Forensic Science*. New York: Facts On File, 2004. This encyclopedic work covers most of the important general concepts in forensic science at a level that is understandable to the general reader.

De Forest, Peter R., E. E. Gaensslen, and Henry C. Lee. *Forensic Science: An Introduction to Criminalistics*. New York: McGraw Hill, 1983. Although this book is now somewhat outdated, it is a classic textbook in the field of forensic science, well worth the attention of any beginning student in the field.

Fisher, Barry A. J. *Techniques of Crime Scene Investigation*, 7th edition. Boca Raton, Fla.: CRC Press, 2003. This book is an upper-level textbook used in police academies, colleges, and universities that contains advanced descriptions of a variety of essential forensic technologies.

Fuller, Charlie. *Forensic Science: Crime and Detection*. Broomall, Pa.: Mason Crest, 2004. This short book provides a good general introduction to forensic science for the young adult reader.

Genge, Ngaire E. *The Forensic Casebook: The Science of Crime Scene Investigation*. New York: Ballantine Books, 2002. This book is a readable general introduction to forensic science techniques written for high school and general adult readers.

Inman, Keith, and Norah Rudin. *Principles and Practice of Criminalistics: The Profession of Forensic Science*. Boca Raton, Fla.: CRC Press, 2001. One of the classics in the field of criminalistics, this book provides an excellent general introduction to the principles of forensic science as well as the field of criminology as a profession.

James, Stuart H., and Jon J. Nordby, eds. *Forensic Science*, 2nd edition. Boca Raton, Fla.: CRC Press, 2005. This introductory textbook in forensic science covers the range of technologies available in the field.

Morton, James. *Catching the Killers: A History of Crime Detection*. London: Ebury Press, 2001. This popular history of six major tools used in forensic science—fingerprinting, ballistic analysis, offender profiling, infiltrators and surveillance, interrogation, and DNA typing—was written as a companion to a popular BBC Two series on the history of forensic science.

Saferstein, Richard. *Criminalistics: An Introduction to Forensic Science*, 9th edition. Upper Saddle River, N.J.: Prentice Hall, 2006. This widely popular textbook on forensic science has chapters on the technology of fingerprint analysis, DNA typing, and other forensic techniques, with a useful general introduction to the field of criminalistics.

Thorwald, Jürgen. *The Century of the Detective*. New York: Harcourt, Brace & World, 1964. In this classic work on forensic science, the author focuses on a number of important cases through which forensic science became a respected and widely used tool of law enforcement.

Tilstone, William J. *Forensic Science: An Encyclopedia of History, Methods, and Techniques*. Santa Barbara, Calif.: ABC-CLIO, 2004. As the title suggests, this reference work covers essentially all of the most important features of the forensic sciences.

FINGERPRINTING

BOOKS

Ashbaugh, David R. *Quantitative-Qualitative Friction Ridge Analysis: An Introduction to Basic and Advanced Ridgeology*. Boca Raton, Fla.: CRC

Press, 1999. This technical treatise on the analysis of ridge patterns in fingerprints includes an excellent history on the development of the technology.

Beavan, Colin. *Fingerprints: The Origins of Crime Detection and the Murder Case That Launched Forensic Science.* New York: Hyperion, 2001. This fascinating history of the early development of fingerprint technology also has additional information on other related forensic techniques, especially that of anthropometry.

Champod, Christophe, Chris J. Lennard, Pierre Margot, and Milutin Stoilovic. *Fingerprints and Other Ridge Skin Impressions.* Boca Raton, Fla.: CRC Press, 2004. This work provides a comprehensive review of the scientific basis of fingerprint identification techniques with an extended discussion of the methodology involved in those techniques. The book is of special interest because it attempts to respond to recent concerns about the scientific basis of fingerprint evidence in criminal cases.

Cole, Simon A. *Suspect Identities: A History of Fingerprinting and Criminal Identification.* Cambridge, Mass.: Harvard University Press, 2001. The author offers a fascinating history of fingerprinting that emphasizes its original functions in British colonial India and the United States, where it was used to classify Chinese immigrants. Cole discusses relatively recent problems in the use of the technique caused by poorly trained examiners and problems with some fingerprint technologies that has led to its replacement, in many instances, by DNA typing.

Collins, Clarence Gerald. *Fingerprint Science: How to Roll, Classify, File, and Use Fingerprints.* Incline Village, Nev.: Copperhouse Publishing Company, 2001. The author provides an introduction to the technique of fingerprint taking that is suitable for anyone with no experience in the field.

Cowger, James F. *Friction Ridge Skin: Comparison and Identification of Fingerprints.* Boca Raton, Fla.: CRC Press, 1993. This work provides an introduction to the theory and practice of the taking, interpreting, and comparing of fingerprints.

Faulds, Henry. *Dactylography, or the Study of Fingerprints.* Halifax: Milner & Company, [1912]. Faulds's book is one of the earliest texts on fingerprinting and is now a classic in the field. Also available online at http://galton.org/fingerprints/books/faulds/faulds1912dact1upclean.pdf.

———. *Guide to Fingerprint Identification.* Stoke on Trent, U.K.: Wood, Mitchell and Co., 1905. Also available online at http://galton.org/fingerprints/books/faulds/faulds1905guide1up.pdf.

Gaensslen, R. K., and Henry C. Lee, eds. *Advances in Fingerprint Technology*, 2nd ed. Boca Raton, Fla.: CRC Press, 2001. This book is an updated version of one of the standard works on fingerprint technology, originally published in 1991. The chapters are written by experts in the field who discuss the latest developments in fields such as identification of latent prints, fingerprint identification with ninhydrin, automated fingerprint identification and imaging systems, and measurement of fingerprint individuality.

Galton, Francis. *Fingerprints*. Amherst, N.Y.: Prometheus Books, 2006. This edition is a reprint of one of the classics in the field of fingerprinting, first published by Galton in 1892. Also available online at http://galton.org/books/fingerprints/index.htm.

Henry, E. R. *Classification and Uses of Fingerprints*. London: Routledge, 1900. Also available online at http://galton.org/fingerprints/books/henry/henry1900classification1up.pdf.

Herschel, Sir William. *The Origin of FingerPrinting*. London: Oxford University Press, 1916. Also available online at http://galton.org/fingerprints/books/herschel/herschel1916origins1up.pdf.

Jain, Lakhmi C., Ugur Halici, Isao Hayashi, S.B. Lee, and Shigeyoshi Tsutsui, eds. *Intelligent Biometric Techniques in Fingerprint and Face Recognition*. Boca Raton, Fla.: CRC Press, 1999. This review of the latest developments in fingerprint technology also contains an introduction to the new and growing field of face-recognition technology as a means of personal identification.

Jones, Gary W. *Introduction to Fingerprint Comparison*. Temecula, Calif.: Staggs Publishing, 2000. The author describes the fundamental and essential features of fingerprint comparison for beginners with little or no previous experience in the field.

Komarinski, Peter. *Automated Fingerprint Identification Systems (AFIS)*. San Diego: Academic Press, 2004. Said to be the "first comprehensive title" on this subject, the book is well written, easily understood, and comprehensive with a good discussion of the history of automated fingerprint identification systems, a review of the way in which they work, and how they have been implemented thus far.

Leighton, Lallie D., Sally A. Schehl, Yvette E. Trozzi, and Colleen Wade, eds. *Processing Guide for Developing Latent Prints*. Washington, D.C.: Latent Print Unit, Federal Bureau of Investigation, 2000. This work is a standard manual on the collection, development, and interpretation of latent fingerprints.

Maltoni, Davide, Dario Maio, Anil K. Jain, and Salil Prabhakar. *Handbook of Fingerprint Recognition*. New York: Springer Verlag, 2003. This technical work deals with the basic principles of fingerprinting, fingerprint sensing, fingerprint analysis and representation, fingerprint matching, fingerprint classification and indexing, synthetic fingerprint generation, other biometric systems, fingerprint individuality, and securing fingerprint systems.

Ratha, Nalini, and Ruud Bolle, eds. *Automated Fingerprint Identification Systems*. New York: Springer Verlag, 2003. The articles in this collection provide a review of the history of fingerprint recognition systems and a discussion of systems now in use and standards that have been developed for the technology. The book is intended for professionals in the field and researchers.

Sengoopta, Chandak. *Imprint of the Raj: How Fingerprinting Was Born in Colonial India*. London: Macmillan, 2003. This exhaustive study reviews the events that led to the use of fingerprinting by members of the British government in its dealings with the native population of India.

Tuthill, Harold. *Individualization: Principles and Procedures in Criminalistics*. Salem, Ore.: Lightning Powder, 1994. The author provides an excellent overall introduction to the general principles and procedures that underlie the identification of individuals involved in crimes.

U.S. Department of Justice. *The Science of Fingerprints: Classification and Uses*. Washington, D.C.: Federal Bureau of Investigation. U.S. Department of Justice, [2002]. This latest revision of a book originally published in 1973 provides a broad overview of the principles and techniques involved in fingerprint analysis. Early editions of the book are also available through Project Gutenberg at http://www.gutenberg.org/files/19022/19022h/19022h.htm.

ARTICLES

Acree, Mark A. "*People v. Jennings:* A Significant Case in American Fingerprint History." *The Print*, vol. 14, no. 4, July–August 1998, pp. 1–2. The author discusses a case from 1911 when fingerprints were used to convict Thomas Jennings of the murder of Clarence Hiller. In that case, the Illinois Supreme Court recognized that "standard authorities on scientific subjects discuss the use of fingerprints as a system of identification, concluding that experience has shown it to be reliable." Based on this decision, Jennings was convicted of the murder.

Ashbaugh, D. R. "Poroscopy." *The Print*, vol. 11, no. 6, November–December 1995, pp 1–7. This article describes the history and technology of poroscopy, the use of pores in the hands and fingers as a means of forensic identification. Although the technique is rarely used today, it continues to be of some historical interest to those who work with fingerprinting.

Benedict, Nathan. "Fingerprints and the Daubert Standard for Admission of Scientific Evidence: Why Fingerprints Fail and a Proposed Remedy." *Arizona Law Review*, vol. 46, no. 3, 2004, pp. 519–549. The author reviews the history of fingerprinting as a forensic tool, discusses current questions about its validity, and recommends changes that would allow the use of fingerprinting with greater confidence in criminal trials.

Berg, Eric. "Digital Enhancement and Transmission of Latent Prints: Who Will Set the Standards?" *The Print*, vol. 12, no. 4, July–August 1996, pp. 6–9. The author raises questions about maintaining the integrity of identification techniques when working with digital images of fingerprints rather than the prints themselves.

Berry, John, and David A. Stoney. "History and Development of Fingerprint." In Henry C. Lee and R. E. Gaensslen, eds. *Advances in Fingerprint Technology*. Boca Raton, Fla.: CRC Press, 2001. The introductory chapter to this collection of articles deals with a general review of the early history of fingerprinting as a forensic tool.

Bradford, Russell R. "Mary E. Holland: America's First Fingerprint Instructor." *The Print*, vol. 14, no. 5, September–October 1998, pp 1–2. The author provides a brief biographical sketch of the first person in the United States to offer regular instruction in fingerprint analysis.

Clark, J. D. D. "ACEV: Is It Scientifically Reliable and Accurate?" *Journal of Forensic Identification*, vol. 52, no. 4, 2002, pp. 401–408. The author considers the most common method of fingerprinting—Analysis, Comparison, Evaluation, and Verification—and asks how reliable and valid it is in a court of law. He concludes that "it is scientifically and biologically impossible for two persons to have twelve or more Galton detail in sequence," justifying the use of fingerprints.

Cole, Simon A. "Is Fingerprint Identification Valid? Rhetorics of Reliability in Fingerprint Proponents' Discourse." *Law & Policy*, vol. 28, no. 1, January 2006, pp. 109–135. The author points out that few or no validation studies for the use of fingerprinting as valid forensic evidence exist and that, given the existence of legal precedent *(Daubert v. Merrell Dow Pharmaceuticals)* allowing the admission of such evidence in legal proceedings, there is little motivation to conduct such studies.

———. "More than Zero: Accounting for Error in Latent Fingerprint Identification." *Journal of Criminal Law & Criminology*. vol. 95, no. 3, 2005, pp. 985–1,078. The author analyzes a number of well-known cases in which fingerprint analysis was shown to be incorrect and argues that "We need to acknowledge that latent print identification is susceptible to error, like any other method of source attribution, and begin to confront and seek to understand its sources of error."

———. "What Counts for Identity? The Historical Origins of the Methodology of Latent Fingerprint Identification." *Science in Context*. vol. 12, no. 1, Spring 1999, pp. 139–172. The author discusses two parallel traditions for fingerprinting in forensic science, one of which is based on a scientific hypothesis that no two prints are exactly alike, and another that focuses on the practical need to use fingerprints for identification purposes in criminal cases. He explains how these two traditions have recently collided as court challenges to the scientific tradition have begun to appear.

Epstein, Robert. "Fingerprints Meet Daubert: the Myth of Fingerprint "Science" Is Revealed." *Southern California Law Review*, vol. 75, no. 3, 2002, pp. 605–657. The article reconsiders and analyzes the long-held belief that fingerprints are an almost insurmountable piece of evidence supporting a prosecution in a criminal trial.

Evett, I. W., and R. L. Williams. "A Review of the Sixteen Point Fingerprint Standard in England and Wales." Published simultaneously in *Fingerprint World*, vol. 21, October 1995, pp. 82–95, and *Journal of Forensic Identification*, vol. 46, January–February, 1996, pp. 1–14 and reprinted in *The Print*, vol. 12, no. 1, January--February, 1996, pp 1–13. Also available online at http://www.scafo.org/library/120101.html. Various law enforcement agencies have adopted different standards for the comparison of fingerprints. In the United States, 12 points of similarity are required for a match; in England and Wales, 16 points. This article reviews the history behind the adoption of that standard in England and Wales.

Faulds, Henry. "On the Skin-Furrows of the Hand." *Nature*, vol. 22, no. 574, p. 605, October 28, 1880. This is one of the historic articles in the history of fingerprinting, in which Faulds describes the general principles of fingerprint analysis and his use of the technique in two cases. The article has been reprinted in a number of places and is available online in many places also. For example, see http://www.clpex.com/Articles/History/Faulds1880.htm.

"The Fingerprint Controversy." *Issues in Science and Technology*, vol. 20, no. 2, January 2004, pp. 9–13. This discussion among experts about the validity of fingerprint evidence was initiated by an article by Jennifer Mnookin in the September 2003 issue of this journal.

Futrell, Ivan Ross. "Hidden Evidence: Latent Prints on Human Skin." *FBI Law Enforcement Bulletin*, vol. 65, no. 3, April 1996, pp. 21–25. The author discusses special problems of recovering fingerprints left on human skin. Also available online http://www.fbi.gov/publications/leb/1996/aprl1965.txt.

Galton, Sir Francis. "Personal Identification and Description." This monograph is based on a lecture given at the Royal Institution on May 25, 1888, in which Galton describes the history of the development of fingerprinting and the basic principles on which it is based. The monograph has been reprinted in a number of places. See, for example, http://www.scafo.org/library/100801.html.

Geller, B., J. Almog, P. Margot, and E. Springer. "A Chronological Review of Fingerprint Forgery." *Journal of Forensic Sciences*, vol. 44, no. 5, 1999, pp. 963–968. This review discusses 30 instances of fingerprint forgery and the methods used to detect these forgeries.

Grieve, David L. "Daubert and Fingerprints: *The United States of America v. Bryan C. Mitchell.*" *The Sleuth*, vol. 37, no. 1, June 1999, pp. 8–9. Reprinted in *The Print*, vol. 15, no. 4, July–August 1999, pp 3–5, and also available online at http://www.scafo.org/library/150402.html. This article is a good general introduction to and discussion of one of the landmark cases in recent forensic history in the United States.

Henry, Sir E. R. "Fingerprints Found at the Scenes of Crime How to Photograph and Prepare Exhibits for Production in Court." *Classification and Uses of Finger Prints*, 4th edition. London: His Majesty's Stationery Office, 1913, pp. 105–109. This article is of considerable historical interest because it describes the technology of fingerprinting and its status at a very early stage of its use in forensic science by one of the technology's leading experts. The article has been reprinted in *The Print*, vol. 11, no. 3, May–June 1995, pp. 1–3, and is available online at http://www.scafo.org/library/110301.html.

Herschel, William. "Skin Furrows of the Hand." *Nature*, vol. 23, no. 578, November 28, 1880, p. 76. This letter to the journal *Nature* is an important document in the history of fingerprinting. In it Herschel describes his use of fingerprints as a means of identification during his tour of duty in India. Herschel's letter infuriated Faulds, who took it as an attempt to wrest credit for the discovery of fingerprinting from himself. The letter has been reproduced in a number of places. See, for example, http://www.clpex.com/Articles/History/Herschel1880.htm.

Inbau, Fred E. "Scientific Evidence in Criminal Cases. III. FingerPrints and PalmPrints." *Journal of Criminal Law and Criminology*, vol. 25, no. 3, September–October 1934, pp. 500–516. This article is one of a series of three (the others being on ballistic fingerprints and the polygraph) on the scientific basis of some widely used forensic techniques by a well known and highly respected legal expert on the subject.

Kaye, David H. "Questioning a Courtroom Proof of the Uniqueness of Fingerprints." *International Statistical Review*, vol. 71, no. 3, December 2003, pp. 521–533. In response to growing concerns about the validity and reliability of fingerprints as evidence in criminal cases, the U.S. government has introduced as evidence statistical studies affirming the legitimacy of fingerprinting. This article questions the validity of those studies and considers the ongoing problems of fingerprinting as a forensic tool.

Lawson, Tamara F. "Can Fingerprints Lie?: Reweighing Fingerprint Evidence in Criminal Jury Trials." *American Journal of Criminal Law*, vol. 31, no. 3, Fall 2003, pp. 1–66. The author reviews mounting evidence that fingerprint evidence is not as reliable as it has long been thought, and what this change means for the criminal justice system.

Mairs, G. Tyler. "Can Two Identical Ridge Patterns Actually Occur—Either on Different Persons or on the Same Person?" *Finger Print and Identifica-*

tion, vol. 27, no. 4, November 1945. Reprinted in *The Print*, vol. 10, no. 4, April 1994, pp 3–7. Although an old article, it is one that raises one of the most fundamental issues in all of fingerprinting; whether identical fingerprints are or are not possible.

McRoberts, Alan L. “Fingerprints: What They Can and Cannot Do!” *The Print*, vol. 10, no. 7, June 1994, pp. 1–3. Although somewhat dated, this is an excellent general overview of the process of taking fingerprints and the information that can be obtained from prints.

Mnookin, Jennifer L. “Fingerprint Evidence in an Age of DNA Profiling.” *Brooklyn Law Review*, vol. 67, no. 1, 2001, pp. 13–70. The article was written for a symposium on the past, present, and future of DNA profiling and reviews the early history of fingerprinting as a forensic tool. The author compares that history with the early history of DNA typing and examines the question as to how these histories now present practical problems for judges dealing with challenges to the validity of fingerprint identifications.

———. “Fingerprints: Not a Gold Standard: Judges Are Showing Signs of Skepticism, and It’s about Time.” *Issues in Science and Technology*, vol. 20, no. 1, September 2003, 47–54. The author reviews a January 2002 decision by Judge Louis Pollack in *United States v. Llera Plaza*, in which he claims that fingerprinting is not a sufficiently confirmed scientific technology to allow its use in criminal cases.

Olsen, Eobert D., Sr. “A Fingerprint Fable: The Will and William West Case.” *Identification News*, vol. 37, no. 11, November 1987, pp. 8–10. Also available online at http://www.scafo.org/library/110105.html. The author retells one of the most famous stories in the early history of fingerprinting in which authorities at the Leavenworth Federal Penitentiary confused two men, Will and William West, a confusion that was resolved only when fingerprints from the two men were taken.

Pankanti, Sharath, Salil Prabhakar, and Anil K. Jain. “On the Individuality of Fingerprints.” *IEEE Transactions on PAMI*, vol. 24, no. 8, August 2002, pp. 1010–1025. The authors attempt to develop a scientific method for predicting the likelihood that the minutiae in any two fingerprints will be identical and come up with a number of conclusions about the reliability of fingerprint evidence, primarily that “(i) contrary to the popular belief fingerprint matching is not infallible and leads to some false associations, (ii) the performance of automatic fingerprint matcher does not even come close to the theoretical performance, and (iii) due to the limited information content of the minutiae-based representation, the automatic system designers should explore the use of non-minutiae based information present in the fingerprints.”

Risinger, D. Michagel, and Michael J. Saks. “A House with No Foundation: Forensic Science Needs to Build a Base Rigorous Research to Establish

Its Reliability." *Issues in Science and Technology*, vol. 20, no. 1, Fall 2003, pp. 35ff. The authors point out that a number of scientific tests, such as fingerprinting and polygraph testing, are based on very shaking scientific foundations and that scientists need to develop more robust evidence for the validity and reliability of such tests.

Skipper, Leigh M., and Robert Epstein. "Just How Reliable Is Fingerprint Evidence?" *The Liberty Legend*, vol. 1, no. 10, May 2000, pp. 2–3. Also available online at http://www.clpex.com/Information/USvMitchell/RobertEpstein/AFD_newsletter_EpsteinLeigh_p2&3.pdf. Two defense attorneys review the recent increase in interest in testing the validity and reliability of fingerprint evidence spurred by the case of *U.S. v. Mitchell.*

Sombat, Jessica M. "Latent Justice: Daubert's Impact on the Evaluation of Fingerprint Identification Testimony." *Fordham Law Review*, vol. 70, no. 6, May 2002, pp. 2819–2868. The author discusses some effects of the *Daubert* case on the use of fingerprint evidence in criminal trials.

Specter, Michael. "Do Fingerprints Lie?" *New Yorker*, May 27, 2002, pp. 96–105. This extended review of recent cases in which fingerprint evidence has come into question also includes an analysis of the validity and reliability of the long-honored system of making personal identifications.

Steele, Lisa J. "The Defense Challenge to Fingerprints." *Criminal Law Bulletin*, vol. 40, no. 3, 2004, pp. 213–240. The author raises the question as to how a defense attorney can respond to fingerprint evidence that appears to indict his or her client. Her response is that such evidence is neither foolproof nor fraud proof and should be viewed with the same amount of skepticism as any other piece of evidence.

Stoney, David A. "Fingerprint Identification: Scientific Status." In D. L. Faigman, D. H. Kaye, M. J. Saks, and J. Sanders, eds. *Modern Scientific Evidence: The Law and Science of Expert Testimony*, 2nd ed., vol. 2, St. Paul, Minn.: West Publishing, 2002, pp. 368–399. This article provides a comprehensive analysis of the current state of fingerprinting as a forensic tool based on the ongoing debate that arose because of the case of *U.S. v. Mitchell.*

Zabell, Sandy L. "Fingerprint Evidence." *Journal of Law and Policy*. vol. 13, no. 1, 2005, pp. 143–179. The author makes a powerful argument that there is no scientific basis for the argument that fingerprints are unique and that they can, therefore, not be used as an infallible method of identification. He points in particular to the problems of identifying latent versus inked fingerprints. He argues that the most serious problem with fingerprint analysis today is that forensic scientists have no true understanding of the actual error rate in analyzing fingerprints.

Annotated Bibliography

REPORTS

National Institute of Standards and Technology. "NIST Image Group's Fingerprint Research." Information Access Division, National Institute of Standards and Technology. Available online. URL: http://www.itl.nist.gov/iad/894.03/fing/fing.html. This web page contains a number of documents developed by the NIST's Image Group dealing with scientific aspects of fingerprinting. Some of the topics for which reports are available are the automated fingerprint identification system, the development of algorithms for use on rolled fingerprint impressions, the development of algorithms for use on latent fingerprints, comparative performance of classification methods for fingerprints, and neural network fingerprint classification.

United States General Accounting Office. *INS Fingerprinting of Aliens: Efforts to Ensure Authenticity of Aliens' Fingerprints: Report to Congressional Requesters*. Washington, D.C.: General Accounting Office, [1994]. This report was prepared at the request of Congress by the General Accounting Office and reviews the legislative basis for fingerprinting of aliens, current practices, and technology involved in the process.

WEB DOCUMENTS

Acree, Mark A. "What Is Science? The Dilemma of Fingerprint Science Revisited." SCAFO online articles. Available online. URL: http://www.scafo.org/library/140403.html. Accessed on March 25, 2007. The author discusses the characteristic features to decide whether fingerprint analysis can be considered a truly scientific discipline. He decides that it is and explains why.

Berg, Erik C. "Legal Ramifications of Digital Imaging in Law Enforcement." *Forensic Science Communications*, vol. 2, no. 4, October 2000. Available online. URL: http://www.fbi.gov/hq/lab/fsc/backissu/oct2000/berg.htm. Accessed on March 25, 2007. This article offers an intensive and extensive analysis of the legal issues involved in the use of digital imaging of fingerprints for law enforcement agencies.

Budowle, Bruce, JoAnn Buscaglia, and Rebecca Schwartz Perlman. "Review of the Scientific Basis for Friction Ridge Comparisons as a Means of Identification: Committee Findings and Recommendations." *Forensic Science Communications*. vol. 8, no. 1, January 2006. Available online. URL: http://www.nlada.org/Defender/forensics/for_lib/Documents/1135190260.95/2006_01_research02.htm. As the result of an incorrect identification of a latent fingerprint at the FBI laboratory, the agency commissioned a study by three senior members of the scientific staff to review the scientific basis of fingerprint identifications and to recommend research that would test the underlying hypotheses of fingerprint analysis.

Chesapeake Bay Division, International Association for Identification. "Latent Fingerprint Processing Techniques—Selection & Sequencing Guide." Available online. URL: http://www.cbdiai.org/Reagents/main.html. Accessed on August 21, 2006. This web page offers a very complete description of all the methods available for collecting and interpreting fingerprint patterns.

Clemens, Daryl W. "Fingerprint Evidence." Crime and Clues: The Art and Science of Criminal Investigation. Available online. URL: http://www.crimeandclues.com/fingerprints.htm. Accessed on August 31, 2006. This collection of online articles focuses on the history and background of fingerprint analysis and methods used for collecting and interpreting fingerprints.

Clpex.com. "Complete Latent Print Examination." Complete Latent Print Examination. Available online. URL: http://www.clpex.com/. Accessed on July 26, 2007. This broad-ranging web site provides fundamental information on fingerprinting techniques, a list of consultants, chatboard, summary of recent events involving the use of fingerprint analysis, and guidelines and information on standard fingerprint indexing systems.

CrimTrac. "Fingerprints." Available online. URL: http://www.crimtrac.gov.au/systems_projects_fingerprints.html. Accessed on March 25, 2007. An Australian web site summarizes key dates in the history of fingerprinting and explains the basic principles of fingerprint analysis.

Dechman, Gordon H. "Fingerprint Identification Standards for Emerging Applications." Available online. URL: http://www.ct.gov/dss/cwp/view.asp?a=2349&q=304808. Last modified on October 20, 2005. The author, a specialist at the state of Connecticut's Department of Social Services, provides a good general introduction to the latest technology in fingerprinting.

"Digital Fingerprints." Available online. URL: http://www.eneate.freeserve.co.uk/index.html. Last updated in May 2005. A web site that includes some interesting historical documents on fingerprinting and some technical discussions of methods for capturing and analyzing latent fingerprints.

Dorf, Michael C. "Admitting Error and Admitting Fingerprints: Is There a Sound Factual Basis for the Law?" FindLaw Legal News and Commentary. Available online. URL: http://writ.news.findlaw.com/dorf/20020320.html. Posted on March 20, 2002. The author reviews the decision by federal judge Louis Pollak not to admit fingerprint evidence in a trial over which he was presiding, his later reversal of his own ruling, and the significance of the events for the future of fingerprinting as evidence in criminal trials.

Annotated Bibliography

"Early Fingerprint Pioneers." Available online. URL: http://ridgesandfurrows.homestead.com/early_pioneers.html. Accessed on August 21, 2006. The web site includes abbreviated biographical sketches of important figures in the history of fingerprinting, including William James Herschel, Sir Edward Richard Henry, Henry Faulds, Alphonse Bertillon, and Francis Galton.

Ferriola, Thomas J. "Scientific Principles of Friction Ridge Analysis & Applying Daubert to Latent Fingerprint Identification." Available online. URL: http://www.clpex.com/Articles/ScientificPrinciplesbyTomFerriola.htm. Accessed on March 25, 2007. The author offers a very long discussion of the basics of fingerprinting, along with a review of the history of fingerprinting technology and a review of the current status of fingerprinting as a valid basis of evidence in criminal cases. The article ends with a list of links to cases in which fingerprinting has been challenged in recent court cases.

Fingerprints.TK. "Welcome to the World of Fingerprints." Fingerprints, Vingerafdrukken. Available online. URL: http://www.xs4all.nl/~dacty/. Last updated on June 10, 2006. This web site provides information on virtually every aspect of fingerprint analysis, including articles on incipient ridges, minutiae, patterns, pores, prints on animals, and strange prints. The site also has a valuable FAQ section that answers most of the basic questions about fingerprinting, a discussion group on fingerprinting, ideas for school projects, and current news about fingerprinting.

Geradts, Zeno. "Zeno's Forensic Site." Available online. URL: http://forensic.to/forensic.html. Last updated on May 6, 2006. This web site is divided into four major parts: general information, forensic sciences, forensic medicine, and forensic psychiatry/psychology. The Fingerprints section of forensic sciences has an extensive list of links on the subject.

German, Ed. "Cyanoacrylate (Superglue) Fuming Tips." Superglue Fuming Tips. Available online. URL: http://onin.com/fp/cyanoho.html. Last updated on August 1, 2003. This web site is an excellent source of background information on the use of cyanoacrylate for fingerprinting, methods for its use, a timeline of the development of the technique, and other useful information on the procedure.

———. "The History of Fingerprints." Available online. URL: http://onin.com/fp/fphistory.html. Last updated on June 8, 2006. The author provides a summary of the most important dates and individuals in the history of fingerprinting as a forensic technique.

———. "Latent Print Examination." Available online. URL: http://www.onin.com/fp/. Accessed on July 31, 2006. This very detailed web site contains information on almost every aspect of fingerprinting, with much of the information keyed to the age and professional level of the reader. Many of the topics are classified as expert topics, general information, or investigator topics. The web site also provides access to an online version of Michele Triplett's book, *Fingerprint Terms*, Alex Mankevich's *Online Processing Guide*, and a number of other important resources. The site also has a summary of all of the so-called *Daubert* cases, in which the validity of fingerprint identification has been called into question.

Hanson, Todd. "Researchers Develop Fingerprint Detection Technology." Los Alamos National Laboratory. Available online. URL: http://www.lanl.gov/news/index.php?fuseaction=home.story&story_id=2343. Accessed on September 10, 2006. Researchers from the University of California working at the Los Alamos National Laboratory announce the discovery of a new fingerprinting technology based on a sophisticated method of detecting the elements present in a fingerprint residue.

Harris, Tom. "How Fingerprint Scanners Work." Available online. URL: http://computer.howstuffworks.com/fingerprintscanner.htm. Accessed on October 1, 2006. This article describes automated devices for scanning and interpreting digital fingerprints, with information on recent developments and a discussion of the pros and cons of the technology.

"The History of Fingerprinting in Criminal Identification and the Launch of Forensic Science." Fingerprints. Available online. URL: http://people.stu.ca/~mclaugh/FINGERPRINTS/HISTORICAL_REACTIONS_WEBPAGE/FINGERPRINTS.HTML. Accessed on March 25, 2007. This web site emphasizes the history of fingerprinting in Canada with descriptions of some events of special importance in the country's history of the forensic sciences.

Information Technology Laboratory. Information Access Division. National Institute of Standards and Technology. "Latent Fingerprint Homepage." Available online. URL: http://fingerprint.nist.gov/latent/. Last updated on December 4, 2006. The National Institute of Standards and Technology (NIST) conducts a number of programs related to fingerprint analysis, the most recent of which was a workshop on latent print analysis held in April 2006 that was devoted to the evaluation of automated latent fingerprint algorithms. This web site also has links to other pages dealing with fingerprint issues and other biometric issues. For a summary of NIST's activities in this field, see http://fingerprint.nist.gov/.

Joseph, Linda C., and Linda D. Resch. "Fingerprinting." Available online. URL: http://www.cyberbee.com/whodunnit/fp.html. Accessed on March 25, 2007. A division of the "Who Dunnit?" web site on forensic procedures, this section includes sections on the history of fingerprinting, classification of fingerprints, and methods of fingerprint identification.

Langenburg, Glenn. "Defending against the Critic's Curse." Available online. URL: http://www.clpex.com/Articles/CriticsCurse.htm. Posted in September 2002. This article was written by a practicing latent fingerprint investigator in response to three critics of the validity and reliability of fingerprint evidence, Simon Cole, James Starrs, and David Stoney. The author provides a detailed and extensive response to the arguments offered by each of these three individuals.

"Latent Print Development/Photography Techniques." Available online. URL: http://www.clpex.com/Reference.htm#History. Accessed on March 25, 2007. This section in a long bibliography on fingerprinting is of special interest because it contains a number of links to special types of fingerprint tests, such as the Liquinox solution for processing adhesives for latent prints, Handiprint in postmortem fingerprinting, recovering latent prints on firearms, testing for blood on with amido black, fluorescein as a replacement for luminol, vacuum metal deposition, and fluorescent gentian violet jumper identification.

Latent-prints.com. Available online. URL: http://www.latentprints.com/. Accessed on March 25, 2007. This web site is devoted to "the sharing of articles, ideas, and discussion regarding the impression evidence sciences," that deal primarily with latent fingerprints, latent print examination, and fingerprint identification.

Lennard, Christopher J., and Trevor Patterson. "Dactyloscopy: The Science of Fingerprinting." The Thin Blue Line. New South Wales Police Service. Available online. URL: http://www.policensw.com/info/fingerprints/indexfinger.html#index. Accessed on October 1, 2006. This superb web site covers virtually every aspect of digital fingerprinting, including a history of fingerprinting, fingerprint identification in Australia, friction ridge skin, classification and identification of fingerprints, fingerprint pattern classification, fingerprint patterns, fingerprint identification, latent fingerprints, techniques for fingerprint detection and enhancement, automated fingerprint identification systems, and abbreviations used in fingerprinting.

Lightning Powder Company. "A Brief History of Fingerprinting in the U.S." Available online. URL: http://www.redwop.com/minutiae.asp?action=showArticle&ID=105. Accessed on July 31, 2006. This article provides a brief history of fingerprinting in the United States.

———. "Processing for Latent Prints." Available online. URL: http://www.redwop.com/technotes.asp#2. Accessed on September 10, 2006. In a series of excellent technical notes, the Lightning Powder Company describes how to perform two dozen standard procedures for lifting and identifying fingerprints. Included are both generic tests, such as amido black, basic red 28, basic yellow 40, and crystal violet tests, as well as proprietary tests, such as 3M™ Novec™ Engineered Fluid HFE7100, Small Particle Reagent (SPR), StickySide Powder, and TapeGlo™ Fluorescent Dye.

Louisiana Public Defenders' Association. "Daubert vs. Dow." Available online. URL: http://www.lapda.org/daubert.htm#KUMHO%20TIRE.

Accessed on March 25, 2007. The Louisiana Public Defenders' Association presents an extended discussion of the relevance of the *Daubert* hearing for defense attorneys with a number of detailed links to other sources of information.

McRoberts, Alan. "The Examination of Fingerprints." Southern California Association of Fingerprint Officers. Available online. URL: http://www.scafo.org. Accessed on October 1, 2006. McRoberts, a member of the Los Angeles Police Department, offers a concise and well-written general introduction to the underlying principles and procedures involved in fingerprint examinations.

Meaney, Jim. "Fingerprints: A Historical Timeline." Fingerprint America. Available online. URL: http://www.fingerprintamerica.com/fingerprint-History.asp. Accessed on June 7, 2006. Meaneys present a very lucid and complete review of the major events in the worldwide history of fingerprinting, with special emphasis on important events in the United States.

"Michele Triplett's Fingerprint Terms." Available online. URL: http://fprints.nwlean.net/. Last updated on March 5, 2007. This web site is a superb resource for scientific and historical terms, acronyms, important individuals and organizations, court cases, and other topics related to fingerprinting.

Moenssens, Andre A. "The Reliability of Fingerprint Identification: A Case Report." Forensic-Evidence.com. Available online. URL: http://forensic evidence.com/site/ID/pollak2002.html. Accessed on September 10, 2006. The author discusses and analyzes the decision by a judge to reverse himself on the admissibility of fingerprint evidence, and how the case relates to recent controversy over the reliability of fingerprint evidence.

"Papers by Dr. William Babler." Available online. URL: http://www.clpex.com/Information/Babler/BablerArticles.htm. Accessed on March 25, 2007. This collection of eight scientific papers on the development of skin ridges in the prenatal child summarizes research by one of the world's experts on the topic.

Prabhakar, Salil, and Anil Jain. "Fingerprint Identification." Available online. URL: http://biometrics.cse.msu.edu/fingerprint.html. Accessed on March 25, 2007. Prabhakar and Jain offer a good, general, and brief introduction to the use of fingerprints as a means of identification.

"Ridges and Furrows." Available online. URL: http://ridgesandfurrows.homestead.com/index.html. Accessed on August 21, 2006. One of the best and most complete web sites on fingerprinting available. The site includes extended discussions of a variety of topics, such as "What Is a Fingerprint?," "Early Pioneers," "Scientific Research," "Significant Dates & Events," "Friction Skin Anatomy," "Friction Skin Growth," "Integumentary System," "S.O.C.O. (scene of crime procedures), "Latent Print Development," "Friction Ridge Identification," "'Daubert' Challenges," "Digital Image Technology," and "Education & Training."

Rodriguez, Julia. "South Atlantic Crossings: Fingerprints, Science, and the State in Turn-of-the-Century Argentina." *American Historical Review*, (online version), vol. 109, no. 2, April 2004. Available online. URL: http://www.historycooperative.org/journals/ahr/109.2/rodriguez.html. Accessed on March 28, 2007. The author provides an excellent account of the work of Argentine criminologist Juan Vucetich, with attention to the impact of European developments in anthropometry and fingerprinting.

"Significant Dates and Events." Available online. URL: http://www.ridgesandfurrows.homestead.com/landmark.html. Accessed on June 7, 2006. The web site has a very complete chronology of major events in the history of fingerprinting.

South Wales Police. "'Every Contact Leaves a Trace'—A History of Fingerprinting." South Wales Police Museum. Available online. URL: http://www.southwales.police.uk/fe/master.asp?n1=8&n2=253&n3=1028. Accessed on June 7, 2006. The web site includes an excellent chronology of the history of fingerprinting, with interspersed comments on other forensic techniques, with special emphasis on developments in the United Kingdom and Australia.

"State of Arizona vs. Toribio Rodriguez." Available online. URL: http://www.clpex.com/Information/Starrs/Arizona_v_Rodriguez_Starrs_Testimony.pdf. Accessed on March 25, 2007. A transcript of a very interesting court case in which a critic of fingerprint evidence testifies for the defense and is questioned in detail by the prosecution about his views on fingerprinting.

"SWGFAST: Scientific Working Group on Friction Ridge Analysis, Study And Technology." Available online. URL: http://www.swgfast.org/. Updated April 19, 2006. SWGFAST is an association of experts in the field of fingerprint analysis. It was created in 1995 with the support of the Federal Bureau of Investigation (FBI) to develop standards for the training and certification of fingerprint analysts. This web site contains approved guidelines developed by the organization for the certification of various types of fingerprint examiners and procedures used in the field. The web site also contains an extensive glossary of terms used in the field.

BALLISTIC ANALYSIS

Books

Burrard, Gerald, Major Sir. *The Identification of Firearms and Forensic Ballistics*. London: Herbert Jenkins, 1934. This early and now classic discussion of the origins of ballistic analysis was written by an Englishman who was involved in a number of court cases involving ballistic issues. The book has gone through a number of editions and revisions and was first published in the United States in 1962. Some topics covered in the book are types of firearms; cartridges and their components; ignition, combustion and pressure; ascertaining the range of a fatal shot; time of a fatal shot and other problems; identification of firearms by means of fired cartridge cases; identification of firearms by means of fired bullets; identification of firearms: technique and examples; and identification of the make of firearms.

Davis, John E. *Tool Marks, Firearms and the Striagraph*. Springfield, Ill.: Charles C. Thomas, 1958. A classic in the field, the book describes the use of the striagraph in identifying tool and ballistic marks. The striagraph had been invented in 1938 by J. Howard Matthews and was later refined and improved by Davis.

Gunther, Jack D., and Charles O. Gunther. *The Identification of Firearms*. New York: John Wiley and Sons, 1935. One of the earliest books to discuss in detail the principles involved in the identification of firearms and ammunition, this book spends nearly half of its time on a detailed discussion of ballistic issues in the Sacco and Venzetti case of 1927.

Hatcher, Julian S. *Textbook of Firearms Investigation, Identification and Evidence*. Plantersville, S.C.: Small-Arms Technical Publishing Co., 1935. This work is probably the first textbook on the subject of ballistics analysis, written by an officer of the U.S. Army who had spent more than two decades in design, manufacturing, and testing of ammunition and firearms. Hatcher's book received widespread praise from his colleagues and was adopted as an instructional tool at many police academies and other educational facilities. He produced an updated version of the book with J. A. C. Weller in 1957 under the same title.

Hatcher, Julian S., Frank J. Jury, and Jac Weller. *Firearms Investigation, Identification and Evidence*, 3rd ed. Harrisburg, Pa.: Stackpole Books, 1977. This book is the updated version of one of the classic texts on the identification of firearms and ammunition.

Heard, Brian J. *Handbook of Firearms and Ballistics*. Chichester, England: John Wiley & Sons, 1997. This text provides a broad review of the types of firearms available in countries around the world along with a description of methods for identifying weapons and ammunition used in crimes.

Matthews, J. Howard. *Firearms Identification*. 3 vols. Springfield, Ill.: Charles C. Thomas, 1962. This comprehensive review of the subject is now somewhat outdated, but still of interest from a historical and basic background standpoint.

Warlow, Tom. *Firearms, the Law, and Forensic Ballistics*. Boca Raton, Fla.: CRC Press, 2nd ed., 2005. This book is probably one of the most thorough and complete texts on ballistic analysis currently available. The author has worked for more than 40 years in the United Kingdom in a variety of law enforcement positions, and his book has something of a British emphasis. One portion of the book is devoted to a review of the beginnings of ballistic analysis; the history of firearms legislation in Great Britain, the United States, and the European Union; and the presentation of criminal evidence in courts of law. By far the greatest focus of the book, however, is on the technical aspects of ballistic analysis, with discussions of microscopic analysis of markings, features of internal and external ballistics, terminal and wound ballistic characteristics, methods of examination of ballistic evidence, and proof marks and proof of firearms. Although filled with technical information, the book is readily accessible to the nonspecialist.

ARTICLES

Biasotti, Alfred A. "A Statistical Study of the Individual Characteristics of Fired Bullets." *Journal of Forensic Science*, vol. 34, no. 1, 1959, pp. 34–50. Based on the author's doctoral thesis, the study reported in this article is one of the most comprehensive examinations of the properties of bullets fired from guns ever conducted.

———, and John Murdock. "The Scientific Basis of Firearms and Toolmark Identification." In D. L. Faigman, et al., eds. *Modern Scientific Evidence.* San Francisco, Calif.: West Law, San Francisco, 1997. This article provides a general discussion of the theoretical basis and experimental background for the use of toolmarks and firearms markings in criminal investigations by two experts in the field.

Cook, C. W. "Ballistics and the Firearms Examiner," *AFTE Journal*, vol. 10, no. 2, June 1978, pp. 49–51. Cook offers a good introductory and general discussion of the principles of ballistics analysis.

Goddard, Colonel C. H. "A History of Firearms Identification to 1930." *AFTE Journal*, vol. 30, no. 3, pp. 225–265. This extensive review of the early history of firearms identification was written by one of the pioneers in the field.

Inbau, Fred E. "Scientific Evidence in Criminal Cases. I. Firearms Identification. "Ballistics" *Journal of Criminal Law and Criminology*, vol. 24, no. 4, November–December 1933, pp. 825–844. One of a series of three articles (the others being on fingerprinting and the polygraph) on the scientific basis of some widely used forensic techniques that was written by a well known and highly respected legal expert on the subject.

Lott, John R., Jr. "Bullets and Bunkum." *National Review*, vol. 54, November 11, 2002, pp. 26+. This general review of efforts to pass ballistic fingerprinting laws on the federal and state levels was written by a frequent critic of such laws.

Nosanchuk, Matt, and Stephen P. Hallbrook. "Symposium: Does the United States Need a Database for National Ballistic Fingerprints?" *Insight on the News*, November 26, 2002, pp. 46–49. The authors offer a pro and con discussion about the usefulness and feasibility of developing a ballistic fingerprinting system for weapons in the United States.

REPORTS

George Washington University. PollingReport.com. "Guns(p. 2)." Available online. URL: http://www.pollingreport.com/guns2.htm. Accessed on March 25, 2007. This report provides a summary of a number of public opinion polls taken between 1999 and 2003 on the question of gun control in general and the use of ballistic fingerprinting in particular.

Kopel, David B., and H. Sterling Burnett. "Ballistic Imaging: Not Ready for Prime Time." National Center for Policy Analysis. Policy Backgrounder No. 160, April 30, 2003. Available online. URL: http://www.ncpa.org/pub/bg/bg160. The authors offer an extensive review of ballistic fingerprinting with an explanation of the procedures involved; an analysis of ballistic databases, their successes and failures, advantages and disadvantages; a review of the Maryland and New York ballistic fingerprinting laws and of the California Bureau of Forensics's study on ballistic fingerprinting; and conclusions as to the likely success of ballistic databases.

Thompson, Robert M., Jerry Miller, Martin G. Ols, and Jennifer C. Budden. *Ballistic Imaging and Comparison Of Crime Gun Evidence*. Washington, D.C.: National Integrated Ballistic Information Network Program, Bureau of Alcohol, Tobacco and Firearms, U.S. Department of the Treasury, May 13, 2002. This report concerns the National Integrated Ballistic Information Network Program, an automated system for comparing bullet and cartridge casing markings in the identification of weapons used in crimes. The report was prepared in response to a request by the state of California to comment on its own report on ballistic databases. The report points out that the bureau's Integrated Ballistic Identification System (IBIS) is significantly less effective in identifying weapons that previous reports have found. It discusses some fundamental issues involved in the use of IBIS by state and local law enforcement agencies.

Tobin, John J., Jr. "MD-IBIS Progress Report #2: Integrated Ballistics Identification System." Pikesville, Maryland, September 2004. Available online. URL: http://doubletap.cs.umd.edu/~purtilo/ibis.pdf. This report was prepared by the Maryland State Police as required by the 2000 act establishing a ballistic database for use in ballistic fingerprinting in the state. The report concludes that the program has been almost entirely without value.

Tulleners, Frederic A. "Technical Evaluation: Feasibility of a Ballistics Imaging Database for All New Handgun Sales." Sacramento, Calif.: Sacramento and Santa Rosa Criminalistics Laboratories, Bureau of Forensic Services, California Department of Justice, October 5, 2001. Available online. URL: http://www.nssf.org/PDF/CA_study.pdf. This document reports on a classic study on ballistic fingerprinting undertaken to determine the feasibility of creating a ballistic fingerprinting law in California similar to those passed in Maryland and New York. The study concludes that a ballistic database would probably not be feasible for the state for a variety of reasons.

U.S. Department of Justice, Office of the Inspector General, Audit Division. "The Bureau of Alcohol, Tobacco, Firearms and Explosives' National Integrated Ballistic Information Network Program." Audit Report 05-30. Washington, D.C.: U.S. Department of Justice, June 2005. This report is a 163-page summary of the history, features, and accomplishments of the National Integrated Ballistic Information Network (NIBIN) program conducted to determine whether "(1) the NIBIN program has been fully deployed with the capability to compare ballistic images on a national level; (2) controls are adequate to ensure that all bullets and cartridge casings collected at crime scenes and from testfires of crime and (3) ballistic images of bullets and cartridge casings from newly manufactured, imported, or sold firearms are entered into NIBIN, in violation of the Firearm Owners' Protection Act of 1996."

Web Documents

Berg, Stanton O., "Reminiscences of The Pre And Early AFTE Years," Association of Firearm and Tool Mark Examiners. Available online. URL: http://www.afte.org/AssociationInfo/a_berghistory.htm. Accessed on June 23, 2006. This article describes the events that led to the formation of the Association of Firearm and Tool Mark Examiners and the early years of the organization's existence.

Brady Campaign to Prevent Gun Violence. "Ballistic Fingerprints Help Solve Crimes." Available online. URL: http://www.bradycampaign.org/facts/issues/?page=ballistic. Accessed on March 25, 2007. Representatives of the Brady Campaign explain why ballistic fingerprinting can be a useful tool in solving violent crimes and offers a response to the "gun lobby's myths" on the subject.

Chan, Jeff. "The Sight." Available online. URL: http://www.sightm1911.com/lib/tech/fingerprint.htm. Last updated on January 9, 2004. This collection of web-based articles and reports is designed for use "in countering the 'ballistic fingerprinting' lies" made by proponents of ballistic fingerprinting laws.

Doyle, Jeffrey Scott. "FirearmsID.com." Available online. URL: http://www.firearmsid.com/new_index.htm. Accessed on August 31, 2006. Doyle's web site contains useful information on virtually every aspect of firearms identification, including pages on distance determination, case profiles, the history of firearms identification, the use of gelatin in identification procedures, a general introduction to ballistics, firearms safety, a collection of articles of general interest, a firearms forum, a resource center, information on expert testimony, and a classroom and help desk on firearms identification.

Hamby, James E. "The History of Firearm and Toolmark Identification." *AFTE Journal*, vol. 31, no. 3, Summer 1999. Available online. URL: http://www.firearmsid.com/A_historyoffirearmsID.htm. This well-written and comprehensive review of the history of firearm and toolmark identification, written by the director of Marion County (Indiana) Forensic Services Agency since 1985, divides the topic into chronological periods that clearly show the evolutionary development of ballistic analysis in the United States and other nations.

Internet Pathology Laboratory for Medical Education. "Ballistics." Available online. URL: http://medlib.med.utah.edu/WebPath/TUTORIAL/GUNS/GUNBLST.html. Accessed on October 1, 2006. A very detailed and well presented discussion of the basics of ballistics. The web page is a section of Firearms Tutorial, which is part of the Internet Pathology Laboratory for Medical Education operated by the Florida State University College of Medicine, intended for students and workers in the health care sciences studying pathology.

Introduction to Firearms Identification, An. "Fundamentals of Firearms ID." FirearmsID.com. Available online. URL: http://www.firearmsid.com/A_FirearmsID.htm. Accessed on July 31, 2006. This web page provides an excellent introduction to the methods available for identifying weapons and ammunition, and contains good illustrations of the equipment that is used and some samples of identifications that have been made.

Long, Duncan. "The Myth of Ballistic Fingerprinting." Available online. URL: http://duncanlong.com/sciencefictionfantasyshortstories/ballisticfingerprints.htm. Posted on October 26, 2002. This essay is written by "an internationally recognized firearms expert" explaining why plans to do ballistic fingerprinting on all guns is an unrealistic concept.

Lott, John R. Jr. "Ballistic Fingerprinting's a Dud: Another Failed Guncontrol Strategy." National Review Online. Available online. URL: http://www.nationalreview.com/comment/lott200502040751.asp. Posted on February 04, 2005. Lott reviews the efforts in Maryland and New York state to implement ballistic fingerprinting programs and attempts to explain why such programs have failed.

Magnusson, Paul. "Ballistics Fingerprinting: A Waste of Time." BusinessWeek Online. Available online. URL: http://www.businessweek.com/bwdaily/dnflash/oct2002/nf20021024_9610.htm. Posted on October 24, 2002. The author argues that ballistic databases have virtually no chance of success in contributing to efforts to find and prosecute the perpetrators of violent crime. The article is a response to an article in favor of ballistic fingerprinting by Lorraine Woellert in the same issue of the online magazine.

Malecki, Tracy. "New Forensic Technology Facilitates Tracing Bullets and Cartridge Cases." *The Compiler* (newsletter of the Illinois Criminal Justice Information Authority). Available online. URL: http://www.icjia.state.il.us/public/index.cfm?metaSection=Publications&metapage=CPLfall9804 Accessed on January 3, 2007. Malecki's well-written article describes the technology of ballistic fingerprinting and discusses its potential applications in forensic science.

Online NewsHour. "Tracking Firearms." PBS NewsHour with Jim Lehrer. Available online. URL: http://www.pbs.org/newshour/bb/law/julydec02/ballistics_1018.html. Posted on October 18, 2002. This report is a transcript of a NewsHour program about the technology of ballistic fingerprinting and the feasibility of ballistic databases between two experts in the field on either side of the latter question.

Ramsland, Katherine. *Ballistics: The Science of Guns*. (ebook) Criminal Mind/Forensics and Investigation. Available online. URL: http://www.crimelibrary.com/criminal_mind/forensics/ballistics/. Accessed on September 10, 2006. Ramsland offers a simplified introduction to ballistic analysis that begins with reviews of the Sacco and Vanzetti case and the St. Valentine's Day massacre, with a discussion of the principles underlying ballistic analysis, and concluding with a discussion of the murder of pornographer Jim Mitchell.

Schehl, Sally A. "Firearms and Toolmarks in the FBI Laboratory." *Forensic Science Communications*. Available online URL: http://www.fbi.gov/hq/lab/fsc/backissu/april2000/schehl1.htm. Accessed on July 26, 2007. The author discusses the use of ballistic fingerprinting by the Federal Bureau of Investigation (FBI) and describes the operation of its ballistics fingerprinting laboratory.

Tartaro, Joseph P. "Ballistic 'Fingerprint' Scheme Far from a Magic Wand." *The New Gun Week*. Available online. URL: http://www.saf.org/pub/rkba/hindsight/HS040100.htm. Accessed on July 26, 2007. The editor of the gun-oriented newsletter outlines the reasons that laws requiring ballistic testing of all guns are not likely to work as adherents expect.

Webster, Daniel W. "Comprehensive Ballistic Fingerprinting of New Guns: A Tool for Solving and Preventing Violent Crime." Available online. URL: http://www.jhsph.edu/gunpolicy/ballistic_fingerprinting.pdf. Updated on

November 21, 2002. The author, director of the Johns Hopkins Center for Gun Policy and Research of the Johns Hopkins Bloomberg School of Public Health, discusses the role of ballistic databases in solving crimes and argues that the apparent lack of success of existing New York and Maryland laws mandating such databases is a result of the lack of a national law that would require a federal database.

Woellert, Lorraine. "Ballistic Fingerprinting: A Lifesaver." BusinessWeek Online. Available online. URL: http://www.businessweek.com/bwdaily/dnflash/oct2002/nf20021024_3210.htm. Posted on October 24, 2002. The author argues that the use of ballistic evidence in solving the so-called Beltway sniper cases shows that the technology is very useful in identifying weapons used in crimes and that the next step should be the development of a national ballistics database. The article is written in conjunction with an article in the same online magazine by Paul Magnusson arguing that ballistic databases are unlikely to accomplish the ends for which they are created.

www.gunowners.com. "Why Ballistic Fingerprinting Is Not an Effective Crime Tool." Available online. URL: http://www.gunowners.org/fs0203.htm. Posted in May 2003. A web site written by and for gun owners provides an annotated list of reasons that the fingerprinting of guns would not reduce gun-related crimes.

ANTHROPOMETRY

BOOKS

Beavan, Colin. "In a Criminal's Bones." In *Fingerprints—The Origins of Crime Detection and the Murder Case That Launched Forensic Science*. New York: Hyperion, 2001. Although the focus of this book is on the history of fingerprinting, the author provides an interesting chapter on anthropometry also.

Bertillon, Alphonse. *Alphonse Bertillon's Instructions for Taking Descriptions for the Identification*. New York: AMS Press, 1989. This text is a reprint of an 1887 manual written by Bertillon on the methodology involved in taking anthropometric measurements.

Hecht, Jennifer Michael. "Careers in Anthropology and the Bertillon Family." In *The End of the Soul: Scientific Modernity, Atheism, and Anthropology in France*. New York: Columbia University Press, 2003. Hecht's chapter offers an interesting and detailed discussion of the Bertillon family, their ethos and lives, along with a description of Alphonse Bertillon's development of anthropometry.

Rhodes, Henry T. F. *Alphonse Bertillon, Father of Scientific Detection*. London: Abelard-Schuman, 1956. Republished by Greenwood Press, 1968. Rhodes's book is one of the few biographies of the founder of anthropometry.

Wallace, Irving. *Monsieur Bertillon.* New York: Fawcett Publications, 1950. Wallace's book is probably the first complete biography in English of Alphonse Bertillon, founder of anthropometry.

Articles

Alden, C. H. "The Identification of the Individual." *American Anthropologist*, vol. 9., no. 14, September, 1896, pp. 295–310. This article is no longer generally available, but an excellent precis can be found on the Anthropology Journal Archive Project web site at http://www.publicanthropology.org/Archive/Aa1896.htm. The article describes the application of anthropometry by the U.S. Army primarily for the identification of deserters and dishonorably discharged soldiers.

Bayle, Edmond. "The Scientific Detective." *American Journal of Police Science*, vol. 2, no. 2, March–April 1931, pp. 158–170. [This article also appears as a chapter in the book *The Underworld of Paris*, by Alfred Morain (E. P. Dutton & Company, 1931)]. The author was successor to Bertillon as director of the French Service de l'Identité Judiciaire. He describes the origin of anthropometry by Bertillon and the current status of the practice in France.

Deflem, Mathieu. "Technology and the Internationalization of Policing: A Comparative-Historical Perspective." *Justice Quarterly*, vol. 19, no. 3, 2002, pp. 453–475. This article provides an excellent discussion of the development of anthropometry in France, its spread to the rest of Europe and the United States, and its eventual demise in favor of fingerprinting.

Fosdick, Raymond B. "The Passing of the Bertillon System of Identification." *Journal of the American Institute of Criminal Law and Criminology*, vol. 6, no. 3, September 1915, pp. 363–369. Fosdick's article was written on the occasion of Alphonse Bertillon's death. It reviews his work on the development of anthropometry and explains why the system "probably suffered its final blow" as a result of his death.

Joseph, Anne M. "Anthropometry, the Police Expert and the Deptford Murders: The Contested Introduction of Fingerprinting for the Identification of Criminals in Late Victorian and Edwardian Britain." In Jane Caplan and John Torpey, eds. *Documenting Individual Identity: The Development of State Practices in the Modern World.* Princeton, N.J.: Princeton University Press, 2001, pp. 165–183. The author discusses the transition in forensic science from anthropometry to fingerprinting and the greater significance of this change in the way of viewing individual identities.

Kaluszynski, Martine. "Republican Identity: Bertillonage as Government Technique." In Jane Caplan and John Torpey, eds. *Documenting Individual Identity: The Development of State Practices in the Modern World.* Princeton, N.J.: Princeton University Press, 2001, pp. 123–138. The author discusses the development of anthropometry as an element in the French government's efforts to keep track of and control its population.

Sekula, Alan. "The Body and the Archive." *October*, vol. 39, Winter 1986, pp. 3–64. The author reviews the development of anthropometry and discusses how the technique proved useful to the French government for the identification of both criminals and other "undesirables" and how other governments have sought the use of such techniques for similar purposes ever since.

Weidgley, Emma Seifret, "Adolphe Quetelet: Pioneer Anthropometrist—1796–1874," *Nutrition Today*, April, 1989, pp. 12–16. Weidgley provides a biographical sketch of the founder of the forensic science of anthropometry.

Reports

Gates, Kelly. *The Past Perfect Promise of Facial Recognition Technology*. Urbana, Ill.: Program in Arms Control, Disarmament, and International Security, University of Illinois at Urbana—Champaign, June 2004. This report deals with the potential of face recognition programs as a way of identifying individuals in the war against terrorism in which the author reviews the development of anthropometry and its long-term significance for other systems of body recognition.

Web Documents

"Anthropometry." Online Encyclopedia. Available online. URL: http://encyclopedia.jrank.org/ANC_APO/ANTHROPOMETRY_Gr_avOpwnros_man_.html. Accessed on September 10, 2006. This article on anthropometry first appeared in the 11th edition of the *Encyclopedia Britannica*, published in 1911. It is of special interest because it was written at a time when anthropometry was still being used by many law enforcement agencies throughout the world.

Aufderheide, Keith. "Forensic Science: Chapter 1: Introduction, Overview and Background." Available online. URL: http://www.oglethorpe.edu/faculty/~k_aufderheide/Forensic_Science/Lecture_Notes/Chapter_1_Lecture_Notes.htm. Accessed on March 28, 2007. This relatively brief introduction to the history of anthropometry is part of a course on forensic science.

Breckenridge, Keith. "Towards the Theory of the Biometric State." Available online. URL: http://www.history.ukzn.ac.za/files/sempapers/Breckenridge 2005.pdf. Accessed on March 25, 2007. This seminar paper on biometrics includes an excellent section on anthropometry and its competition with fingerprinting during the late 19th century.

Annotated Bibliography

Brockman, Andreas. "A Visual Economy of Individuals: The Use of Portrait Photography in the Nineteenth-Century Human Sciences." Available online. URL: http://isp2.srv.v2.nl/~andreas/phd/. Accessed on March 28, 2007. This doctoral thesis deals with the use of photographic images in forensic science but devotes considerable attention to the development of anthropometry by Bertillon and its significance within that general context.

Cole, Simon A. "Fingerprint Identification and the Criminal Justice System: Historical Lessons for the DNA Debate." Available online. URL: http://www.ksg.harvard.edu/dnabook/Simon_Cole_(3)_12903.doc. Accessed on September 10, 2006. The author devotes an extended section of this paper to a review of the development of anthropometry and some lessons for the modern-day debate over DNA fingerprinting that can be learned from Bertillon's work.

Cooley, Craig M. "Daubert and Kumho Tire: A Wake Up Call for the Forensic Sciences." Available online. URL: http://www.lawforensic.com/wake_up.htm#_ftnref1. Accessed on March 28, 2007. This long article deals with the significance of two important court cases dealing with the admissibility of scientific evidence and includes an extended discussion of Bertillon's work in the development of anthropometry.

Dugelay, Jean-Luc. "Reconnaissance du Visage." Available online. URL: http://paristic.labri.fr/TUTORIAL/tutorial_BIO_2_PARISTIC_05.pdf. Posted on November 22, 2005. This slide show discusses the use of facial images for the purposes of recognition and has an excellent description of the Bertillon system, its use in France, and its transfer to the United States. It is one of the best readily available sources of information about anthropometry on the Internet.

Ford, Graham. "Historical Fingerprint Events & People." Available online. URL: http://fingerprints.com/_wsn/page12.html. Accessed on March 25, 2007. The author provides a brief biographical sketch of Alphonse Bertillon and the system of anthropometry he invented.

Guardware. "Fingerprint Recognition II: History of Fingerprinting." Available online. URL: http://www.biometrieonline.net/dossiers/technique/empreintes/History_of_Fingerprinting.pdf. Posted in December 2000. This historical sketch contains a brief but useful review of the rise and fall of bertillonage.

Hunt, Megan. "Anthropometry." Available online. URL: http://acad.erskine.edu/facultyweb/smith/ForensicScience/studentpresentations/Anthropometry.ppt. Hunt has developed an excellent slide presentation describing the history and use of anthropometry with illustrations of the devices and documents used in the field.

Moenssens, Andre A. "Alphonse Bertillon and Ear Prints." Available online. URL: http://forensicevidence.com/site/ID/ID_bertillion.html. Accessed on March 25, 2007. This web page contains a selection taken from the author's book *Fingerprint Techniques* on the use of ear measurements by Bertillon in his system of anthropometry.

National Library of Medicine. "Visible Proofs." National Library of Medicine. Available online. URL: http://www.nlm.nih.gov/visibleproofs/galleries/technologies/bertillon.html. Posted on February 16, 2006. This is a fascinating collection of visual images held by the U.S. National Library of Medicine illustrating the origin and use of anthropometry. An excellent verbal description of the technique is provided as captions for the photographs.

Pavlich, George. "The Accusations of Criminal Identity." Available online. URL: http://www.mcgill.ca/files/legaltheoryworkshop/PavlichAccusationsCriminalIdentity.pdf. Accessed on March 25, 2007. This web page contains a draft of an address to a Legal Theory Workshop held at McGill University on November 17, 2006. It includes an excellent review of the rise, development, and eventual demise of Bertillon's system of anthropometry.

Roberts, Chris. "Biometrics." Available online. URL: http://www.ccip.govt.nz/ccippublications/ccipreports/Biometrics.pdf. Posted in November 2005. Roberts provides an excellent overview of the subject of biometrics that contains some interesting dates in the history of anthropometry.

Rodriguez, Julia. "South Atlantic Crossings: Fingerprints, Science, and the State in Turn-of-the-Century Argentina." *American Historical Review*, (online version). Available online. URL: http://www.historycooperative.org/journals/ahr/109.2/rodriguez.html. Accessed on March 28, 2007. This article provides an interesting discussion of the impact of anthropometry on Juan Vucetich's work in Argentina.

Tarbell, Ida M. "Identification of Criminals: The Scientific Method in Use in France." Available online. URL: http://chnm.gmu.edu/courses/magic/plot/bertillon.html. Accessed on March 25, 2007. This web page is a reprint of an article by a famous muckraker journalist of the time published in *McClure's Magazine* in 1894, about Bertillon's system of anthropometry.

Touloumi, Olga. "The Prison of Regina Coeli: A Laboratory of Identity in Post Risorgimento Italy." Available online. URL: http://dspace.mit.edu/bitstream/1721.1/35125/1/71790581.pdf. Accessed on March 28, 2007. This master's thesis includes an interesting section dealing with the introduction of anthropometry to Italy by Bertillon at the First International Congress on Criminal Anthropology in Rome in 1882 and its use thereafter by the Italian law enforcement community.

Vij, Illa. "Alphonse Bertillon." *The Tribune Saturday Plus*, September 25, 1999. Available online. URL: http://www.tribuneindia.com/1999/99sep25/saturday/fact.htm. Accessed on July 26, 2007. This is a general interest article on the life of Alphonse Bertillon with a review of his development of the science of anthropometry.

Watner, Carl. "'Your Papers, Please!' The Origin and Evolution of Official Identity in the United States." Voluntaryist.com. Issue no. 121. Available online. URL: http://www.voluntaryist.com/articles/121a.php. Accessed on September 10, 2006. The author discusses the development of anthropometry within the general construct of the desire of a nation to be able to identify its citizens, with an analysis of the relevance of that philosophy to modern-day efforts to develop modern systems of identification.

POLYGRAPH TESTING

BOOKS

Alder, Ken. *The Lie Detectors: The History of an American Obsession.* San Diego: Academic Press, 2007. The author discusses the early history of the polygraph, focusing in particular on the work of John Larson, August Vollmer, and Leonarde Keeler.

Ansley, Norman, and Gordon L. Vaughan. *Polygraph: Quick Reference Guide to the Law*, 17th ed. Chattanooga, Tenn.: American Polygraph Association, 2002. This important reference includes a summary of state and federal laws and relevant court cases dealing with the admissibility of polygraph data in court cases.

Block, Eugene G. *Lie Detectors: Their History and Use.* New York: David McKay Company, 1977. This now-outdated book is still useful because of its historical information and general background on the polygraph.

Clifton, Charles. *Deception Detection: Winning the Polygraph Game.* Boulder, Colo.: Paladin Press, 1991. Although intended primarily as a way of helping people to protect themselves from polygraph testing, the book provides excellent background information on the history and technology of polygraphs.

Kleiner, Murray. *Handbook of Polygraph Testing.* Burlington, Mass.: Academic Press, 2001. This standard reference in the field of polygraph testing consists of a collection of articles by experts on topics, such as the comparison question test, the guilty knowledge test, the pre-test interview, the use of the polygraph in personnel screening, countermeasures in polygraph testing, and legal issues in the use of polygraph testing in the United States.

Lykken, David E. *A Tremor in the Blood: Uses and Abuses of the Lie Detector.* New York: Plenum Publishing, 1981, 1998. An expert in polygraph testing reviews the history of lie detection methods and the polygraph and its strengths and weaknesses. He proposes an alternative method of lie detection called the guilty knowledge test as a possible alternative to traditional polygraph testing.

Matte, James Allan. *Forensic Psychophysiology Using the Polygraph: Scientific Truth Verification–Lie Detection*. Williamsville, N.Y.: J.A.M. Publications, 1996. The publisher describes this book as "the long awaited bible of scientific truth verification and lie detection" needed by attorneys, judges, law enforcement personnel, probation and parole officers, forensic psychophysiologists, defendants, litigants, psychologists, researchers, historians, business persons, employers and employees, and various educational institutions.

Segrave, Kerry. *Lie Detectors: A Social History*. Jefferson, N.C.: McFarland & Company, 2003. Segrave's book is an excellent, complete history of the development of concepts behind lie detection, as well as the evolution of polygraphs themselves.

Williams, Douglas Gene. *How to Sting the Polygraph*. Chickasha, Okla.: Sting Publications, 2001. This book guarantees to show a person how to pass a polygraph test.

ARTICLES

Adler, Ken. "A Social History of Untruth: Lie Detection and Trust in Twentieth-Century America." *Representations*, no. 80, Autumn 2002, pp. 1–33. The author examines the somewhat peculiar situation that polygraph testing has reached in the United States, in which the procedure is widely used for a variety of purposes and generally trusted by the general public, although abundant evidence suggests that its results are of only marginal value.

Aftergood, Steven. "Polygraph Testing and the DOE National Laboratories." *Science*, vol. 290, no. 5493, November 3, 2000, pp. 939–940. The author argues that mandated polygraph testing for federal employees "has arguably diminished both science and security at the weapons labs of Los Alamos, Livermore, and Sandia National Laboratories," and explains why that is the case.

Beardsley, Tim. "Truth or Consequences: A Polygraph Screening Program Raises Questions about the Science of Lie Detection." *Scientific American*, vol. 281, no. 4, October 1999, pp. 21, 24. The author reviews charges of espionage at the Los Alamos National Laboratory, the Department of Energy's decision to require polygraph testing as a result of that event, and the evidence about the validity and reliability of polygraph testing.

Bunn, Geoffrey C. "The Lie Detector, Wonder Woman and Liberty." *History of the Human Sciences*, vol. 10, no. 1, January 1997, pp. 91–119. Bunn's article provides a biography of William Moulton Marston with a discussion of his invention of the lie detector and its impact on contemporary forensic science and society in general.

Fiedler, Klaus, Jeannette Schmid, and Teresa Stahl. "What Is the Current Truth about Polygraph Lie Detection?" *Basic and Applied Social Psychology*, vol. 24, no. 4, pp. 313–324. This article reports on a study conducted in response to the German Supreme Court's decision not to accept polygraph results in penal procedures. The authors apply "standard criteria of scientific validity" to assess the most commonly used and influential polygraph procedure, the Control Question Test, and find that the test does not meet, nor even attempt to meet, fundamental standards of internal consistence, reliability, and validity. The authors conclude that "a fair and responsible appraisal of polygraph testing should clearly reveal this lack of validity."

Furedy, John J. "The North American Polygraph and Psychophysiology: Disinterested, Uninterested, and Interested Perspectives." *International Journal of Psychophysiology*, vol. 21, nos. 2–3. February–March 1996, pp. 97–105. Also available online at http://psych.utoronto.ca/~furedy/napoly.htm. The author argues that the group of scientists best qualified to assess the validity and reliability of polygraph testing—psychophysiologists—has largely ignored the topic, permitting people with a vested interest in promoting the technology with an open field for encouraging the wider use of polygraph testing, and without a sound scientific basis for the technology.

Gallai, David. "Polygraph Evidence in Federal Courts: Should It Be Admissible?" *American Criminal Law Review*, vol. 36, no. 1, Winter 1999, pp. 87–116. The author reviews reasons that he thinks evidence obtained from polygraph testing should not be admissible in a court of law.

Grubin, Don, and Lars Madsen. "Lie Detection and the Polygraph: A Historical Review." *Journal of Forensic Psychiatry and Psychology*, vol. 16, no. 2, June 2005, pp. 357–369. Grubin and Madsen offer an excellent review of the history of the polygraph, with a review of controversies surrounding its use and some modern applications.

Honts, Charles R. "The Emperor's New Clothes: Application of Polygraph Tests in the American Workplace." *Forensic Reports*, vol. 4, 1991, pp. 91–116. The author explains that polygraph testing in the private sector has been greatly reduced as a result of the Employee Polygraph Protection Act (EPPA) of 1988, but such testing continues unabated within the federal government, where it is commonly used to detect security risks. The problem is that there is no scientific basis for the tests, and studies have shown that polygraph testing uncovers no more than about 2 percent of guilty subjects who are tested, largely as the result of effective countermeasures used by such individuals.

———. "The Psychophysiological Detection of Deception." *Current Directions in Psychological Science*, vol. 3, no. 3, June 1994, pp. 77–82. The author suggests that progress is being made in developing a scientific basis for polygraph testing, but that "a great deal of research" is still needed before polygraph testing will be a truly useful tool in the detection of deception. Until that research is completed, he suggests that the use of polygraph testing be limited.

Honts, Charles R., Robert L. Hodes, and David C. Raskin. "Effects of Physical Countermeasures on the Physiological Detection of Deception." *Journal of Applied Psychology*, vol. 70, no. 1, February 1985, pp. 177–187. Researchers trained subjects to deceive polygraph testers by a variety of methods such as biting their tongues and pressing their foot against the floor. The experimenters concluded that people "can be trained to defeat a CQT [control question test] in a laboratory paradigm."

Iacono, William G. "Forensic 'Lie Detection': Procedures without Scientific Basis." *Journal of Forensic Psychology Practice*, vol. 1, no. 1, 2001, pp. 75–86. The author discusses the scientific validity of the control question test (CQT), the most common type of polygraph test conducted, and concludes that, due to "serious methodological problems" that characterize research in the field, it is impossible to determine an accurate validity rate for the procedure. He points out that members of the Society for Psychophysiological Research and fellows of the American Psychological Association "hold negative views" about the CQT procedure.

Iacono, William G., and David T. Lykken. "The Validity of the Lie Detector: Two Surveys of Scientific Opinion." *Journal of Applied Psychology*, vol. 82, no. 3, 1997, pp. 426–433. The authors surveyed members of two professional organizations with expertise in the area of lie detection, the Society for Psychophysiological Research and fellows of the American Psychological Association's Division 1 (General Psychology). They received high rates of response (91 percent and 74 percent, respectively) and found that the majority of respondents believe that polygraphic lie detection "is not theoretically sound, claims of high validity for these procedures cannot be sustained, the lie test can be beaten by easily learned countermeasures, and polygraph test results should not be admitted into evidence in courts of law."

Inbau, Fred E. "Scientific Evidence in Criminal Cases. II. Methods of Detecting Deception." *Journal of Criminal Law and Criminology*, vol. 24, no. 6, March–April 1934, pp. 1140–1158. This is one of a series of three articles (the others being on fingerprinting and ballistic fingerprinting) on the scientific basis of some widely used forensic techniques by a well-known and highly respected legal expert on the subject.

Kleinmuntz, Benjamin, and Julian J. Szucko. "Lie Detection in Ancient and Modern Times: A Call for Contemporary Scientific Study." *American*

Psychologist. vol. 39, no. 7, July 1984, pp. 766–776. The authors claim that psychologists have largely ignored polygraph testing, "a technique that is seen as clearly within their purview," a problem because the technique is so inaccurate that it "yields unacceptably high error rates that have had ruinous effects on the lives of many misclassified truthful persons."

———. "On the Fallibility of Lie Detection." *Law & Society Review*. vol. 17, no. 1, 1982, pp. 85–104. The author argues that since "lying does not produce a measurable physiological response" the theoretical basis underlying lie detection systems and devices is "questionable."

MacLaren, Vance. "Can We Trust Counterintelligence Polygraph Tests?" *Polygraph*, vol. 29, no. 2, 2000, pp. 151–155. The author reviews the use of polygraph testing by the U.S. government and concludes that "[c]urrent polygraph security screening procedures make a valuable contribution to the maintenance of national security."

Menges, Paul M. "Ethical Considerations of Providing Polygraph Countermeasures to the Public," *Polygraph*, vol. 31, no. 4, 2002, pp. 254–262. The author, a polygraph examiner for the federal government, argues for the continued use of polygraph testing to promote federal security. He says that "[p]olygraph is scientifically valid and a tremendous investigative tool available to law enforcement and security personnel of this country." He also discusses efforts by "a vocal minority" to eliminate the use of polygraph testing that "run counter to the best interests of society and public safety." In particular, he castigates those who promote the idea of teaching countermeasures to people who are to undergo polygraph testing "by alerting the public to these efforts that aid guilty parties who threaten society, public safety, and quite possibly our national security." See also the response to this article by George W. Maschke in "A Response to Paul M. Menges Regarding the Ethical Considerations of Providing Polygraph Countermeasures to the Public," February 25, 2003. Available online at: http://antipolygraph.org/articles/article029.shtml

Talbot, Margaret. "Duped." *The New Yorker*, July 2, 2007, pp. 52–61. The author describes and discusses a new approach to lie detection, No Lie MRI, that uses brain scans to detect falsehoods. The article includes an excellent review of the development of polygraphy and an assessment of its validity.

Trovillo, Paul V. "A History of Lie Detection." *American Journal of Police Science*, vol. 29, no. 6, March–April 1939, pp. 848–881 and vol. 30, no. 1, May–June 1939, 104–119. This article is probably one of the best available historical reviews of the history of lie detection methods available at the time of writing. Even today, the articles contain information not available in any other source readily available to the general public.

REPORTS

Barland, G. H., C. R. Honts, and S. D. Barger. *Studies of the Accuracy of Security Screening Polygraph Examinations*. Report No. DoDPI89R0001. 1989. Fort McClellan, Ala.: U.S. Department of Defense Polygraph Institute. This report covers what is reputedly the largest study on polygraph accuracy ever conducted. It showed that most innocent individuals submitted to polygraph testing were shown to have answered questions honestly and were, therefore, identified as innocent, while only about a third of guilty individuals were identified as being guilty by the tests. The federal agencies sponsoring the tests decided not to publish the results of the study in the open literature.

BPS Working Party. *A Review of the Current Scientific Status and Fields of Application of Polygraphic Deception Detection*. Leicester, England: British Psychological Society, October 6, 2004. Also available online at http://www.bps.org.uk/downloadfile.cfm?file_uuid=9081F97A306E1C7FB65E570A3444FF4D&ext=pdf#search=%22%22Polygraph%20admissibility%3A%20Changes%20and%20challenges%22%22. This report describes a scientific study that covers the following topics: What is the polygraph? What constitutes a good psychometric procedure? Polygraph testing in criminal investigations; polygraph testing in employment and security screening; the use of the polygraph in the clinical setting; other possible methods to detect deception; and human rights and codes of conduct.

Committee to Review the Scientific Evidence on the Polygraph; Board on Behavioral, Cognitive, and Sensory Sciences and Committee on National Statistics; Division of Behavioral and Social Sciences and Education; National Research Council; National Academies of Science. *The Polygraph and Lie Detection*. Washington, D.C.: The National Academies Press, 2003. This report comes from a committee appointed to "conduct a scientific review of the research on polygraph examinations that pertains to their validity and reliability, in particular for personnel security screening." The report offers a number of conclusions and recommendations, one of the most interesting of which is that the results produced by polygraph testing appear to be overestimated.

Cumming, Alfred. "Polygraph Use by the Department of Energy: Issues for Congress." Washington, D.C.: Congressional Research Service. Available online. URL: http://www.fas.org/irp/crs/RL31988.pdf. Updated October 1, 2003. This report from the Congressional Research Service was requested when a difference of opinion about the usefulness of polygraph testing developed within the Department of Energy. In the report, the Congressional Research Service lays out three options for Congress to consider vis-à-vis use of the polygraph for employee screening: Make polygraph testing more focused, encourage additional research on polygraph accuracy, and discontinue use of polygraph testing for employment testing.

Joint Security Commission. "Redefining Security: A Report to the Secretary of Defense and the Director of Central Intelligence." Washington, D.C.: Joint Security Commission, February 28, 1994. Available online. URL: http://www.fas.org/sgp/library/jsc/chap4.html. Accessed on August 21, 2006. This report was issued by a committee appointed to investigate existing security protocols used in the federal government and to recommend changes that would make such protocols more effective. Chapter 4 of the report discusses the use of polygraph testing and gives the technology "lukewarm" support.

'Lectric Law Library. "ACLU Briefing Paper Number 4." Available online. URL: http://www.lectlaw.com/files/emp28.htm. Accessed on October 1, 2006. This document is a copy of a briefing paper by the American Civil Liberties Union no longer available on the ACLU web site. The paper discusses legal and privacy issues related to the use of polygraph testing for hiring and employment purposes, with a number of recommendations for individuals and organizations using or considering the use of the polygraph.

Office of the Assistant Secretary of Defense. *Polygraph Program: Annual Polygraph Report to Congress*, Fiscal Year 2000. Also available online at http://www.fas.org/sgp/othergov/polygraph/dod2000.html. This extensive report on the use of polygraph testing was prepared by the Department of Defense. It includes data on the number of tests conducted, the number of individuals who failed, and the number who passed. The report also discusses training procedures for polygraph examiners and recent research in the field.

Office of the Assistant Secretary of Defense. *Polygraph Program: Annual Polygraph Report to Congress*, Fiscal Year 2001. Also available online at http://www.fas.org/sgp/othergov/polygraph/dod2001.html. This annual report was prepared by the Department of Defense. It summarizes the department's use of polygraph testing in a variety of settings, describes training and qualification standards for examiners employed by the department, and reviews recent research on polygraph testing.

Polygraphs and Security. A Study by a Subpanel of Sandia's Senior Scientists and Engineers. Sandia, New Mexico, October 21, 1999. Also available online at http://www.fas.org/sgp/othergov/polygraph/sandia.html. This report was prepared by a group of senior scientists at one of the Department of Energy's national laboratories. It concludes that there is very little scientific support for the accuracy of polygraphs and that their use in employee screening may actually increase risks posed by national security because it will be easier for subversives to gain employment, talented workers may be driven away, valuable resources will be wasted on correcting polygraph errors, and employee commitment may be reduced.

Scientific Validity of Polygraph Testing: A Research Review and Evaluation. Washington, D.C.: Office of Technology Assessment, OTATMH15, November 1983. One of the most complete studies of polygraph testing ever conducted, the report finds that there is almost no credible scientific evidence to support the use of polygraph testing for personnel security screening, and that the practice carries with it some serious risks for misuse of the practice by screeners and subjects.

WEB DOCUMENTS

APAOnline. "The Truth About Lie Detectors (aka Polygraph Tests)." Available online. URL: http://www.psychologymatters.org/polygraphs.html. Accessed on July 28, 2007. The American Psychological Association discusses the issue of polygraph reliability and validity and concludes that "[m]ost psychologists agree that there is little evidence that polygraph tests can accurately detect lies."

Bonsor, Kevin. "How Lie-Detectors Work." Available online. URL: http://people.howstuffworks.com/liedetector.htm. Accessed on October 1, 2006. Bonsor provides a clear explanation of the way polygraphs work, the kind of work that polygraphers do, some uses of polygraph testing, and controversies surrounding the technology.

Carroll, Robert Todd. "Polygraph (Lie Detector)." The Skeptics Dictionary. Available online. URL: http://skepdic.com/polygrap.html. Updated on August 19, 2006. Carroll offers an overview of the technology of polygraph testing, its reliability and validity, and reasons for its widespread use. The web site also contains links to other useful sources of information on polygraph testing.

Cops, Inc. "The History and Basic Facts of Polygraph." Cops, Inc.—Polygraph and Investigative Services. Available online. URL: http://www.polygraphexaminer.com/index_files/Page559.htm. Accessed on September 17, 2006. This web site provides a general introduction to the history of the polygraph, along with an explanation of the principles and technology behind its use.

Decker, Ron. "Leonarde Keller." The Polygraph Museum. Available online. URL: http://www.lie2me.net/thepolygraphmuseum/id12.html. Accessed on September 17, 2006. Decker offers a biography of Leonarde Keeler with a detailed description of the polygraph machines that he designed and built.

Fisher, Jim. "The Polygraph and the Frye Case." Jim Fisher. The Official Web Site. Available online. URL: http://jimfisher.edinboro.edu/forensics/frye.html. Last updated on February 24, 2004. The author of the web page presents a detailed discussion and analysis of one of the most famous legal cases relating to the use of the polygraph in forensic science, *Frye v. United States*, decided in 1923.

Global Polygraph. "About the Polygraph." Available online. URL: http://www.globalpolygraph.com.au/works.html. Accessed on June 13, 2006. The web page provides a broad general introduction to the polygraph, its technology, and its uses.

Lafayette Instrument Company. "History." Lafayette Instrument Company. Available online. URL: http://www.globalpolygraph.com.au/works.html. Accessed on September 17, 2006. This commercial web page offers an excellent and unusually complete and detailed history of the development of polygraph testing.

Marin, Jonathan. "He Said, She Said." Available online. URL: http://users.rcn.com/jonmarin/Polygraph1.htm. Accessed on August 31, 2006. Marin suggests a third approach to the use of polygraphs (in addition to use or no use) that involves pairing the results of two tests and an analysis of the scientific, legal, and social issues raised by such an approach.

Maschke, George W., and Gino J. Scalabrini. "The Lie Behind the Lie Detector." Available online. URL: http://www.antipolygraph.org/pubs.shtml. Accessed on July 28, 2007. AntiPolygraph.org, 2005. This web page provides perhaps the most extensive and comprehensive analysis of polygraph testing available on the Internet. The document examines in detail the validity of polygraph testing, government policy on the use of polygraphs, scientific evidence on polygraph examinations, countermeasures that can be used against polygraph testing, and grievance procedures available for use against polygraph policies and use. The report includes a number of case studies relating to each of these aspects of polygraphy.

McCarthy, Susan. "The Truth about the Polygraph." Salon. Available online. URL: http://archive.salon.com/health/feature/2000/03/02/polygraph/. Posted on March 2, 2000. McCarthy offers a description of the history of the polygraph and the way it works, with discussion as to its reliability and possible advantages it may have beyond simply testing the veracity of an individual.

"The Polygraph Place." Available online. URL: http://www.polygraphplace.com/. Accessed on October 10, 2006. The Polygraph Place provides a vast amount of useful information for anyone interested in polygraphy, including explanations as to how a polygraph works and lists of polygraph examiners, schools, associations, equipment, and insurance.

Ramsland, Katherine. *The Polygraph* (ebook). Available online. URL: http://www.crimelibrary.com/forensics/polygraph. Accessed on July 26, 2007. One of Ramsland's ebooks on forensic science, *The Polygraph* offers a general overview of the science of lie detection, with chapters on history of the polygraph, how polygraphs are used, problems with polygraph use, and polygraph applications. The book also contains a good, if somewhat abbreviated, bibliography.

Richardson, Drew C. "Opening Statement on Polygraph Screening of Supervisory Special Agent Dr. Drew C. Richardson, FBI Laboratory Division, before the United States Senate Committee on the Judiciary Subcommittee on Administrative Oversight and the Courts on the 29th day of September, 1997." Available online. URL: http://antipolygraph.org/hearings/senatejudiciary1997/richardsonstatement.shtml. Accessed on October 1, 2006. FBI agent Richardson testifies that polygraph testing is "completely without any theoretical foundation and has absolutely no validity." Moreover, he points out that almost anyone can be taught how to respond in such a way as to make a polygraph test useless for identifying true and false statements.

Singel, Kati. "The Polygraph: The Modern Lie Detector." Available online. URL: http://www.umw.edu/hisa/resources/Student%20Projects/Singel/students.umw.edu/_ksing2os/polygraph/origin.html. Accessed on July 1, 2006. Singel offers a detailed analysis of the history of lie detection with special emphasis on the use of polygraph testing and its impact on law enforcement in the United States and screening of military personnel.

Stein, Jeff. "Lies, Damned Lies and Polygraphs." Salon. Available online. URL: http://www.salon.com/april97/news/news970410.html. Posted on April 10, 1997. The author argues that "'Tea leaves and witchcraft' are keeping hundreds of qualified, innocent people out of government jobs." He explains the operation of polygraphs and the reasons they cannot be trusted to get the truth in many instances.

Stone, LeRoy A. "Using the Polygraph to Detect Lying and Deception: The Hoax of the Century." *Electronic Journal of Forensic Psychonomics.* Available online. URL: http://www.home.earthlink.net/~lastone2/forensicarticle6.htm. Accessed on January 24, 2007. Stone, who has worked in the field of forensic criminal psychology for many years, provides a review of the history of polygraph testing. He offers some interesting first-hand experiences about the use of polygraphs in lie detection and explains why he calls the machine "the hoax of the century."

Zaid, Mark S. "Polygraph Letter." Available online. URL: antipolygraph.org/hearings/senate-judiciary-2001/zaid-letter.shtml#_ftn1. Accessed on July 28, 2007. This letter is written by a member of SourceWatch, a project of the Center for Media and Democracy, as a follow-up to his testimony before the Senate Judiciary Committee hearing on Issues Surrounding the Use of Polygraphs, held on April 25, 2001. He concludes with the observation that "[t]here is something inherently wrong and unfair with the current federal polygraph policies that are implemented throughout the different law enforcement and intelligence agencies of our government. Without intervention by this Committee, there is little chance these policies will ever change."

DNA TYPING

BOOKS

Balding, David J. *Weight-of-Evidence for Forensic DNA Profiles.* New York: John Wiley & Sons, 2006. This book is a technical treatise on the statistical analysis of data obtained from DNA testing.

Billings, Paul R. *DNA on Trial: Genetic Identification and Criminal Justice.* Plainview, N.Y.: Cold Spring Harbor Laboratory Press, 1992. This text is a collection of papers presented at a conference on DNA typing sponsored by the American Association for the Advancement of Science.

Buckleton, John S., Christopher M. Triggs, and Simon J. Walsh, eds. *Forensic DNA Evidence Interpretation.* Boca Raton, Fla.: CRC Press, 2004. This collection of articles was written by experts in the field on technical questions on the interpretation of DNA evidence.

Budlowe, Bruce, ed. *DNA Typing Protocols: Molecular Biology and Forensic Analysis.* Natick, Mass.: Eaton Publishing Company, 2000. This laboratory manual on DNA typing techniques was compiled by a team from the FBI Forensic Sciences Research and Training Laboratory.

Butler, John M. *Forensic DNA Typing: Biology, Technology, and Genetics of STR Markers*, 2nd ed. Burlington, Mass.: Elsevier Academic Press, 2005. This series of articles describes and discusses the latest development in technical procedures of DNA typing, intended for the advanced or specialized reader.

Carracedo, Angel, ed. *Forensic DNA Typing Protocols.* Totowa, N.J.: Humana Press, 2005. This technical book deals with the methods used in DNA typing and analysis.

Coleman, Howard, and Eric Swenson. "DNA in the Courtroom: A Trial Watcher's Guide." Seattle, Wash.: GeneLex Corp., 1994. Also available online at http://www.genelex.com/paternitytesting/paternitybook.html. This book was originally written as a technical aid for reporters covering the O. J. Simpson trial. It was later expanded to deal more completely with DNA typing and its forensic applications.

Easteal, Simon, Neil McLeod, and Ken Reed. *DNA Profiling: Principles, Pitfalls and Potential.* Boca Raton, Fla.: CRC Press, 1991. This text is one of the earliest books to present a comprehensive and technical approach to DNA typing and some of the issues it raises.

Evett, I. W., and B. S. Weir. *Interpreting DNA Evidence.* Sunderland, Mass.: Sinauer Associates, Inc., 1998. This technical book deals with the statistical basis of DNA typing. It also includes information on interpreting DNA data and the presentation of DNA typing results in court.

Fischer, Eric A., and Nancy Lee Jones. *DNA Identification and Evidence: Applications and Issues.* Huntington, N.Y.: Novinka Books, 2001. This book provides a general introduction to the use of DNA as a means of identifying individuals; some applications to which DNA typing has been put; and some social, legal, and ethical issues raised by the technology.

Fridell, Ron. *DNA Fingerprinting: The Ultimate Identity.* New York: Franklin Watts, 2001. This book provides a general introduction to the subject of DNA typing. It is intended primarily for high school and general readers. In addition to a discussion of the technology involved in DNA typing, the book outlines some interesting applications and some social issues related to the use of the technology.

Kirby, Lorne T., ed. *DNA Fingerprinting: An Introduction.* New York: Oxford University Press, 1990. One of the first books published on the subject of DNA typing, this text describes the technology involved and applications to a variety of fields, including paternity testing, forensic science, medical diagnostics, wildlife poaching, and plant and animal studies.

Kobilinsky, Lawrence, Thomas F. Liotti, and Jamel Oeser-Sweat. *DNA: Forensic and Legal Applications.* Hoboken, N.J.: Wiley-Interscience, 2004. This book is a comprehensive manual on DNA typing that deals with a range of issues from the collection of evidence to the presentation before courts of the results of DNA typing.

Krawczak, Michael, and J. Schmidtke. *DNA Fingerprinting.* 2nd ed. Oxford, U.K.: Bios Scientific Publishers, 1994. *DNA Fingerprinting* is a technical introduction to DNA typing that includes a consideration of legal and ethical issues involved in the use of the technology along with a consideration of possible future applications.

Lazer, David, ed. *DNA and the Criminal Justice System: The Technology of Justice.* Cambridge, Mass.: MIT Press, 2004. This book covers many aspects of DNA typing including a general review of its current uses and future applications, genetic privacy, DNA data banks, privacy rights in the use of databanks, and the use of databanks in law enforcement programs.

Lee, Henry, and Frank Tirnday. *Blood Evidence: How DNA Is Revolutionizing the Way We Solve Crimes.* New York: Perseus Pub., 2003. The lead author was a member of the legal defense team in the O. J. Simpson murder trial. The book provides a general narrative description of the use of DNA typing in legal cases.

Lee, Henry C., and R. E. Gaensslen, eds. *DNA and Other Polymorphisms in Forensic Science.* Chicago: Year Book Medical Publishers, 1990. This early collection of articles about DNA typing and its forensic applications is still of value today.

Levy, Harlan. *And the Blood Cried Out: A Prosecutor's Spellbinding Account of the Power's of DNA to Free or Convict,* reprint edition. New York: Basic Books, 1996. This book was inspired by the O. J. Simpson murder trial in which the defense managed to convince the jury to ignore DNA evidence, with a review of the history and technology of DNA typing and its application in forensic science.

Lincoln, Patrick J. *Forensic DNA Profiling Protocols.* Totowa, N.J.: Humana Press, 1998. This text is a technical work on the methods used in the analysis of DNA samples.

Read, M. M., ed. *Focus on DNA Fingerprinting Research.* Hauppauge, N.Y.: Nova Science Publishers, 2006. This text provides a review of the most recent research in the field of DNA typing.

———. *Trends in DNA Fingerprinting Research.* Hauppauge, N.Y.: Nova Science Publishers, 2005. This advanced text reviews the latest developments in the technology of DNA typing.

Robertson, J., A. M. Ross, and L. A. Burgoyne, eds. *DNA in Forensic Science: Theory, Techniques, and Applications.* New York: Ellis Horwood, 1990. This book offers a comprehensive review of the scientific and technological issues involved in DNA typing and its applications in forensic situations.

Rudin, Norah, and Keith Inman. *An Introduction to Forensic DNA Analysis,* 2nd ed. Boca Raton, Fla.: CRC Press, 2002. This text is an excellent general introduction to the subject of DNA typing with a short review of the history of the technology, a detailed and complete description of the methods involved, and a review of some important legal and social issues related to DNA typing.

———. *Protocols in Forensic Biology: DNA Typing and Physiological Fluid Analysis.* Boca Raton, Fla.: CRC Press, 2007. Designed for professionals in the field, the book provides a comprehensive review of procedures used in the typing of DNA samples.

Scheck, Barry, Peter Neufeld, and Jim Dwyer. *Actual Innocence.* New York: New American Library, 2001. The founders of the Innocence Project offer a number of chilling examples of criminal justice gone awry and tell how DNA typing has helped to save a number of improperly convicted individuals.

Sheindlin, Gerald. *Genetic Fingerprinting: The Law and Science of DNA.* Bethel, Conn.: Rutledge Books, 1996. This book is of special interest, perhaps, because it was written by the judge in one of the early landmark cases involving DNA typing, *People v. Castro.*

Spencer, Charlotte A. *Genetic Testimony: A Guide to Forensic DNA Profiling.* Upper Saddle River, N.J.: Pearson/Prentice Hall, 2004. *Genetic Testimony* is a short general introduction to DNA typing for readers with little or no background in science.

Wall, W. J. *The DNA Detectives.* London: Robert Hale, 2005. Wall provides a general introduction to the subject of DNA typing with information about its historical development, the techniques used, some applications in forensic science, and ethical issues that have arisen as a result of its use in crime detection.

Weir, Bruce S., ed. *Human Identification: The Use of DNA Markers*. Dordrecht, The Netherlands: Kluwer Academic Publishers, 1995. This collection of essays purports to provide a genetic, statistical, and legal basis for the use of DNA evidence in criminal cases.

Yurevitch, Greg, and Shane Quigley. "Genetic Identification: Implications for Society and Crime Scene Investigation," In *Technology and Privacy in the New Millennium*. [no author]. Boulder, Colo.: Ethica Publishing, 2004. Yurevitch and Quigley analyze the impact of DNA typing on various aspects of society, especially the field of criminology.

ARTICLES

Antler, Christine. "A Brief Tour of DNA Fingerprinting." *The Science Creative Quarterly*, issue 2, January–March 2007, p. 1. Also available online at http://www.scq.ubc.ca/?p=250. This article offers a brief, but clear and well-illustrated, explanation of the basic principles of DNA typing.

Aronson, J. D. "DNA Fingerprinting on Trial: The Dramatic Early History of a New Forensic Technique." *Endeavour*, vol. 29, no. 3, September 2005, pp. 126–131. Aronson provides an excellent review of the first two criminal cases in Great Britain in which DNA evidence was used to establish the guilt of individuals responsible for a crime.

Bailey, Ronald. "Unlocking the Cells–Postconviction DNA Testing of Prisoners." *Reason*, January 2000, pp. 50–51. The author offers a commentary on the value of DNA testing to determine the innocence of prisoners who have been wrongly convicted of crimes.

Balazic, J., and I. Zupanic. "Quality Control and Quality Assurance in DNA Laboratories: Legal, Civil and Ethical Aspects." *Forensic Science International*, vol. 103, no. 1, 1999, pp. S1–S5. Balazic and Zupanic raise a number of legal and ethical issues involved in maintaining appropriate laboratory practices in the procedures used in DNA typing.

Balding, D. J. "When Can a DNA Profile Be Regarded as Unique?" *Science & Justice*, vol. 39, no. 4, October–December 1999, pp. 257–260. The article offers a technical analysis of methods for determining the extent to which some given DNA pattern is unique.

Benecke, Mark. "Coding or Non-Coding, That Is the Question." *EMBO Reports*, vol. 3, no. 6, 2002, pp. 498–501. The author points out that most of the technical and legal issues surrounding DNA typing have now been resolved, leaving scientists and nonscientists with decisions as to the ethical issues surrounding the use of the results from DNA fingerprinting.

———. "DNA Typing in Forensic Medicine and in Criminal Investigations: A Current Survey." *Naturwissenschaften*, vol. 84, no. 5, May 1997, pp. 181–188. The article is a somewhat technical, but well-written review of the current status of DNA typing, with a review of relevant technology, a discussion of ethical issues in the use of the results of DNA analyses, and some recent applications of DNA typing.

Berger, Margaret A. "The Impact of DNA Exoneration on the Criminal Justice System." *Journal of Law, Medicine & Ethics*, vol. 34, no. 2, 320–327. The author reviews the use of DNA typing in the exoneration of men and women incorrectly convicted of crimes they did not commit and discusses some general effects this practice may have on attitudes toward the death penalty, the need for strict regulation of DNA testing laboratories, and the services offered by the forensic sciences themselves.

Bernasconi, Andrew C. "Beyond Fingerprinting: Indicting DNA Threatens Criminal Defendants' Constitutional and Statutory Rights." *American University Law Review*, vol. 50, no. 4, April 2001, pp. 979–1037. The article relates the problems raised by obtaining warrants based on genetic information even though no specific individual may be named in the warrant. Does the use of such warrants, especially when they are used to avoid statute of limitations problems, present a civil liberties issue for the person arrested under the warrant?

Cormier, Karen, Lisa Calandro, and Dennis Reeder. "Evolution of DNA Evidence for Crime Solving—A Judicial and Legislative History," *Forensic Magazine*, vol. 2, no. 3, June–July 2005, pp. 15–18. Also available online at http://www.forensicmag.com/articles.asp?pid=45. The authors discuss the early history of DNA typing, its admissibility in court cases, development of DNA databases, and the use of DNA evidence in exoneration of innocent prisoners.

Cronan, John P. "The Next Frontier of Law Enforcement: A Proposal for Complete DNA Databanks." *American Journal of Criminal Law*, vol. 28, no. 1, January 2000, pp. 119–156. The author outlines the power of DNA typing both for locating and convicting criminals and for exonerating those wrongfully convicted of a crime, and he concludes that a national DNA databank should be implemented to increase the efficiency with which DNA typing is used as a crime-fighting tool.

Dawkins, Richard. "Arresting Evidence: DNA Fingerprinting: Public Servant or Public Menace?" *Sciences*, vol. 38, no. 6, November–December 1998, pp. 20–25. Dawkins provides a general introduction to DNA typing for the non-scientist with a discussion of some possible problems in the use of the technology.

Elkins, Lindsy A. "Five Foot Two with Eyes of Blue: Physical Profiling and the Prospect of a Genetics-based Criminal Justice System." *Notre Dame Journal of Law, Ethics, and Public Policy*, vol. 17, no. 1, 2003, pp. 269–305. Elkins argues that DNA evidence provides a vast amount of physical evidence about individuals (such as hair color, sex, height, and race, that could—but is not—being used in the investigation of crimes, resulting in the fact that many guilty persons are not being arrested of, prosecuted for, and being convicted of crimes for which they are responsible.

Elwell, Lynn. "DNA Goes to Court." *Carolina Tips*, vol. 58, no. 4, October 1995, pp. 1–3. Also available online. URL: http://www.carolina.com/tips/95oct/. The author offers a good general introduction to the methods used in DNA typing, a consideration of statistical issues involved in interpreting DNA results, and a classroom activity that introduces the ideas of DNA typing to students.

Fernandez, Holly K. "Genetic Privacy, Abandonment, and DNA Dragnets: Is Fourth Amendment Jurisprudence Adequate?" *Hastings Center Report*, vol. 35, no. 1, January–February 2005, pp. 21–23. The author discusses the legal implications of an increasingly common practice by law enforcement officers of obtaining DNA evidence from a criminal suspect without obtaining traditional warrants that allow them to do so.

Freckelton, Ian. "DNA Profiling : Forensic Science under the Microscope." In Julia Vernon and Ben Selinger, eds. *DNA and Criminal Justice : Proceedings of a Conference Held 30–31 October 1989*. Canberra: Australian Institute of Criminology, 1992. This is an older article that presents a good general summary of the technology of DNA typing and the legal issues raised by its new (at the time) availability, many of which remain significant.

"Genes and Justice." *Judicature*, vol. 83, no. 3, November–December 1999. A special issue of the journal is devoted to genetics-related issues faced by the judicial system, with articles on "Keeping the Gate: The Evolving Role of the Judiciary in Admitting Scientific Evidence," "From Crime Scene to Courtroom: Integrating DNA Technology into the Criminal Justice System," and "Complex Scientific Evidence and the Jury."

Giannelli, Paul C. "Crime Labs Need Improvement: The Quality of the Labs Is Criminal; Government Must Invest in Personnel and Facilities." *Issues in Science and Technology*, vol. 20, no. 1, Fall 2003, pp. 55ff. Although DNA typing is now widely accepted within the scientific and law enforcement communities, a major remaining problem is the care with which testing laboratories carry out the necessary procedures and, hence, the extent to which human error taints the result of DNA testing.

Gohara, Miriam S. "A Lie for a Lie: False Confessions and the Case for Reconsidering the Legality of Deceptive Interrogation Techniques." *Fordham Urban Law Journal*, vol. 33, no. 3, March 2006, pp. 791–842. The author reviews a common procedure within the law enforcement community that allows the police to present suspects with false information in the hope of obtaining a confession and how the new availability of evidence from DNA typing ought to change that practice.

Gosline, Anna. "Will DNA Profiling Fuel Prejudice?" *New Scientist*, vol. 186, no. 2494, April 8, 2005, p. 12. Gosline provides a good review of the

England and Wales National DNA Database (NDNAD), the largest DNA database in the world and some of its forensic successes, along with a discussion of some problems it may pose for non-criminal members of the general public and implications for the suggested expansion of CODIS in the United States.

Grand, Jeffrey S. "The Blooding of America: Privacy and the DNA Dragnet." *Cardozo Law Review*, vol. 23, no. 6, August 2002, pp. 2,277–2,323. The author argues that the collection of DNA samples from suspects may constitute unreasonable search or seizure but acknowledges that there may be circumstances under which such action may be justified when the appropriate protection is provided to the suspect in such cases.

Gross, Samuel R., et al. "Exonerations in the United States, 1989 through 2003." *Journal of Criminal Law & Criminology*, vol. 95, no. 2, Winter 2005, pp. 523–560. The authors review and discuss all cases of exoneration resulting from data derived from DNA typing in the United States between 1989 and 2003.

Haack, Susan. "Trials & Tribulations: Science in the Courts." *Daedalus*, vol. 132, no. 4, Fall 2003, pp. 54–63. Haack provides an analysis of the problems faced by courts when they are confronted with cases that involve scientific issues in which they may not have expertise, with the case of DNA typing as being a particularly strong example.

Hagelberg, Erika, Ian C. Gray, and Alec J. Jeffreys. "Identification of the Skeletal Remains of a Murder Victim by DNA Analysis." *Nature*, vol. 352, no. 6334, August 1, 1991, pp. 427–429. This is one of the classic early papers by a research group led by the founder of the restriction fragment length polymorphism (RFLP) technique for the amplification of small segments of DNA.

Hagerman, Paul J. "DNA Typing in the Forensic Arena." *American Journal of Human Genetics*, vol. 47, no. 5, November 1990, pp. 876–877. The writer of this letter to the editor raises the question as to how human errors during DNA typing may affect the results of DNA evidence presented to the legal system. Also see a follow-up response to this letter at Russell Higuchi, ""Human Error in Forensic DNA Typing," *American Journal of Human Genetics*, vol. 48, no. 6, June 1991, pp. 1,215–1,216.

Harlan, Leigh M. "When Privacy Fails: Invoking a Property Paradigm to Mandate the Destruction of DNA Samples." *Duke Law Journal*, vol. 54, no. 1, October 2004, pp. 179–219. The author points out that the constitutionality of searches for criminal suspects based on evidence obtained from DNA databases has been questioned from a number of angles. He discusses those challenges and suggests a constitutionally more sound way of carrying out such searches.

Herlica, Debra A. "DNA Databanks: When Has a Good Thing Gone Too Far?" *Syracuse Law Review*, vol. 52, no. 3, 2002, pp. 951–977. Does the collection of DNA evidence from individuals who have not been convicted of a crime represent unreasonable search or seizure?

Imwinkelried, Edward J., and D. H. Kaye. "DNA Typing: Emerging or Neglected Issues." *Washington Law Review*, vol. 76, no. 2, April 2001, pp. 413–474. The authors point out that DNA typing has now been widely accepted by all aspects of the law enforcement community, but that many important questions remain to be resolved, including the power of police to collect DNA samples and to use those samples in their investigations, the validity of court orders for the collection of DNA samples, and the permissibility of using DNA samples "abandoned" in public places.

Jeffreys, A. J., J. F. Brookfield, and R. Semeonoff. "Positive Identification of an Immigration Testcase Using Human DNA Fingerprints." *Nature*, vol. 317, no. 6040, October 31–November 6, 1985, pp. 818–819. This is a scientific paper in which the inventor of the restriction fragment length polymorphism (RFLP) technique of DNA typing describes one of the first practical cases in which the technique was used to identify an individual.

Joblin, Mark A., and Peter Gill. "Encoded Evidence: DNA in Forensic Analysis." *Nature Reviews Genetics*, vol. 5, no. 10, October 2004, pp. 739–751. This is an excellent article that provides a historical overview of the development of DNA typing, its methodology, its application in forensic science, and some ethical issues involved in the development of DNA databases.

Jost, Kenneth. "DNA Databases: Does Expanding Them Threaten Civil Liberties?" *CQ Researcher*, vol. 9, no. 20, May 28, 1999, pp. 449–472. This series of articles deals with the background of DNA databases, issues involved in their development and use, the current situation, and future outlook for such databases. A good bibliography is also provided.

Kanon, Diana L. "Will the Truth Set Them Free? No, But the Lab Might: Statutory Responses to Advancements in DNA Technology." *Arizona Law Review*, vol. 44, no. 2, 2002, pp. 449–476. Kanon analyzes laws passed in two states—Illinois and New York—as a result of the growing number of cases in which wrongfully convicted individuals have been exonerated upon the results of DNA evidence that was not available at the time of their trials.

Kaye, D. H. "Bioethical Objections to DNA Databases for Law Enforcement: Questions and Answers." *Seton Hall Law Review*, vol. 31, no. 4, 2001, pp. 936–948. Law enforcement officials and agencies are excited about the promise of DNA databases in solving and prosecuting crimes, but the collection of this highly personal information from individuals poses some serious ethical questions.

———. "The Relevance of 'Matching' DNA: Is the Window Half Open or Half Shut?" *Journal of Criminal Law and Criminology*, vol. 85, no. 3, Winter 1995, pp. 676–695. The author reviews the technology of DNA typing and discusses its admissibility in a court of law.

Kimmelman, Jonathan. "Just a Needlestick Away—DNA Testing Can Convict the Guilty; It Can Also Destroy the Privacy of Millions." *The Nation*, vol. 271, no. 17, November 27, 2000, pp. 17–22. Although laws mandating DNA testing of criminals and DNA databases have value in solving crimes, there is a strong possibility that they may impose too strongly on individuals' civil rights.

Kloosterman, A. D. "Credibility of Forensic DNA Typing Is Driven by Stringent Quality Standards." *Accreditation and Quality Assurance: Journal for Quality, Comparability and Reliability in Chemical Measurement*. vol. 6, nos. 9–10, September 2001, pp. 409–414. The author discusses the importance of ensuring that DNA samples taken for analysis are not contaminated and suggests methods for ensuring that such is the case with samples from which evidentiary DNA is analyzed.

Lindsey, Samuel, Ralph Hertwig, and Gerd Gigerenzer. "Communicating Statistical DNA Evidence." *Jurimetrics*, vol. 43, no. 2, January 2003, pp. 147–163. The authors consider the problem of communicating to courts and juries the meaning of DNA-match probabilities in DNA typing and suggest a "naturalistic" method for doing so in a way that will be understandable and sensible to the target audience.

Luftig, Micah A., and Stephen Richey. "DNA and Forensic Science." *New England Law Review*, vol. 35, no. 3, 2001, pp. 609–613. Luftig and Richey offer an overview of the technical aspects of DNA typing intended for lawyers and students of the law.

Lynch, Michael. "God's Signature: DNA Profiling, the New Gold Standard in Forensic Science." *Endeavour*, vol. 27, no. 2, 2003, pp. 93–97. The author reviews the history of DNA typing and compares the process by which it has been accepted to the acceptance of digital fingerprinting in previous decades.

Lyons, Donna, and Molly Burton. "Proof Positive." *State Legislatures*, vol. 27, no. 6, June 2001, pp. 10–15. The authors analyze the contributions that DNA typing can make to law enforcement programs in several states, with a consideration of the economic, legal, ethical, and other issues posed by the creation of state DNA databases.

Maclin, Tracey. "Is Obtaining an Arrestee's DNA a Valid Special Needs Search Under the Fourth Amendment? What Should (and Will) the Supreme Court Do?" *Journal of Law, Medicine & Ethics*, vol. 34, no. 2, Summer 2006, pp. 165–187. The author discusses privacy issues raised by the use of DNA databases to apprehend criminal suspects who might not be found by traditional forensic means.

Mellon, Jennifer N. "Manufacturing Convictions: Why Defendants Are Entitled to the Data Underlying Forensic DNA Kits." *Duke Law Journal*, vol. 51, no. 3, December 2001, pp. 1,097–1,137. The author describes the process by which many testing laboratories conduct DNA typing tests, making use of special kits designed for that purpose. She points out that technicians may use the kits without really understanding how they are supposed to work, thus producing questionable results for the law enforcement system. She emphasizes the necessity of defense attorneys having access to information about the kits used in producing DNA typing evidence.

Noble, Alice A. "DNA Fingerprinting and Civil Liberties." *Journal of Law, Medicine & Ethics*, vol. 34, no. 2, Summer 2006, pp. 149–152. This essay is an introduction to a special issue of the journal on the subject of DNA typing and civil liberties.

Norton, Amy. "DNA Databases: The New Dragnet." *The Scientist*, vol. 19, no. 7, April 2005, pp. 50–53. As a result of efforts by the administration of President George W. Bush, states are expanding their DNA databases to include a much larger fraction of the population than had been the case in the past. This article explores the reason for this trend and social, ethical, and political questions it may raise about the use of DNA information.

Patton, Stephen M. "DNA Fingerprinting: The *Castro* Case." *Harvard Journal of Law & Technology*. vol. 3, Spring 1990, pp. 223–240. This article is a clearly written review of the technology of DNA typing and a discussion of one of the most important initial cases in which it was used in the United States, *People v. Castro*.

Peterson, Rebecca Sasser. "DNA Databases: When Fear Goes Too Far." *American Criminal Law Review*, vol. 37, no. 3, Summer 2000, pp. 1,219–1,238. Peterson discusses the increasing call for DNA databases, especially among law enforcement agencies, and the civil rights and other issues posed by this growing demand.

Puri, Allison. "An International DNA Database: Balancing Hope, Privacy, and Scientific Error." *Boston College International and Comparative Law Review*, vol. 24, no. 2, 2001, pp. 341–380. The author provides an excellent general review of the history of DNA typing, its scientific basis, and legal issues raised by the creation of DNA databases, especially those with an international component.

Quarmby, Ben. "The Case for National DNA Identification Cards." Duke Law and Technology Review (E-journal), January 1, 2003. Some officials have recommended the development of a national identification card carrying a person's DNA information as a way of protecting against terrorist attacks. This article considers the legal implications of such a proposal.

Reeder, Dennis J. "Impact of DNA Typing on Standards and Practice in the Forensic Community." *Archives of Pathology & Laboratory Medicine*, vol.

123, no. 11, November 1999, pp. 1,063–1,065. Reeder reviews the development of standards and proficiency tests for the procedures used in DNA typing by the FBI's Technical Working Group on DNA Analysis Methods and the National Institute of Standards and Technology.

Reilly, Phil. "Legal and Public Policy Issues in DNA Forensics." *Nature Reviews Genetics*, vol. 2, no. 3, April 2001. pp. 313–317. The author raises questions about the legal and policy issues raised by the increasing popularity of and expansion of DNA databases.

Ritter, Nancy. "Identifying Remains: Lessons Learned from 9/11." *NIJ Journal*, no. 256, January 2007, pp. 20–26. Also available online at http://www.ojp.usdoj.gov/nij/journals/256/lessonslearned.html. Ritter offers an extended review of the use of DNA typing in the identification of people killed during the destruction of the World Trade Center's twin towers on September 11, 2001.

Rosen, Christine. "Liberty, Privacy, and DNA Databases." *The New Atlantis*, no. 1, Spring 2003, pp. 37–52. The author reviews the development of DNA databases with a consideration of some ethical, legal, and other issues raised by their existence and use.

Rothstein, Mark A., and Meghan K. Talbott. "The Expanding Use of DNA in Law Enforcement: What Role for Privacy?" *Journal of Law, Medicine & Ethics*, vol. 34, no. 2, Summer 2006, pp. 153–164. The use of DNA databases by law enforcement officers in the investigation of crimes and the apprehension of suspects raises questions about invasion of the privacy of individuals who may or may not be involved in the investigation.

Saad, Rana. "Discovery, Development, and Current Applications of DNA Identity Testing." *Baylor University Medical Center Proceedings*, vol. 18, no. 2, April 2005, pp. 130–133. Saad reviews the history of DNA typing and its current applications in a variety of fields.

Schneider, P. M. "Basic Issues in Forensic DNA Typing." *Forensic Science International*, vol. 88, no. 1, July 1997, pp. 17–22. The article is a general overview of the technology of DNA typing with some technical, social, and legal questions associated with the technology.

Siegel, Andrew M. "Moving Down the Wedge of Injustice: A Proposal for a Third Generation of Wrongful Convictions Scholarship and Advocacy." *American Criminal Law Review*, vol. 42, no. 4, Fall 2005, pp. 468–492. The author discusses the success of the Innocence Project in exonerating criminals, the general impact this movement has had on the criminal justice in general, and the future impacts that DNA typing may have for incorrectly convicted individuals in the future.

Simoncelli, Tania. "Retreating Justice: Proposed Expansion of Federal DNA Database Threatens Civil Liberties." *Gene Watch*, vol. 17, no. 2, March–April 2004, pp. 3–9. Also available online at http://www.genewatch.org/genewatch/articles/172Simoncelli.html. The author explains how the Advancing Justice through DNA Technology Act of 2003 poses a threat to civil liberties because it significantly increases "the federal government's power to collect, analyze and use information against its own citizens."

Sjerps, M., and A. D. Kloosterman. "Statistical Aspects of Interpreting DNA Profiling in Legal Cases." *Statistica Neerlandica*, vol. 57, no. 3, August 2003, pp. 368–389. The authors deal with some technical statistical problems involved in the presentation of evidence obtained from DNA typing.

Stevens, Aaron P. "Arresting Crime: Expanding the Scope of DNA Databases in America." *Texas Law Review*, vol. 79, no. 4, March 2001, pp. 921–960. The author discusses the problem created by the growing use of DNA typing and the large variability among states in terms of court acceptance of DNA evidence. He argues for the need for a national agency that will set standards for the use of DNA technology in forensic sciences.

Stockmarr, Anders. "Likelihood Ratios for Evaluating DNA Evidence When the Suspect Is Found through a Database Search." *Biometrics*, vol. 55, no. 3, September 1999, pp. 671–677. A problem of considerable interest to forensic scientists and law enforcement officials is to what extent—if at all—DNA evidence obtained from a database versus evidence obtained from a suspect directly and the crime scene may influence estimates of the probability of a match in either case. This article is one of the seminal papers to discuss this point. It was followed by a number of responses and rejoinders in the same and other journals. See, for example, I. W. Evett, L. A. Foreman, and B. S. Weir, "Letter to the Editor," *Biometrics*, vol. 56, no. 4, December 2000, pp. 1274–1276; B. Devlin, "The Evidentiary Value of a DNA Database Search," *Biometrics*, vol. 56, no. 4, December 2000, pp. 1,276–1,277; A. P. Dawid, "Comment on Stockmarr's "Likelihood Ratios for Evaluating DNA Evidence When the Suspect Is Found through a Database Search," *Biometrics* vol. 57, no. 3, September 2001, pp. 976–980; and D. J. Balding, "The DNA Database Search Controversy," *Biometrics*, vol. 58, no. 1, March 2002, pp. 241–244.

Sullivan, K. M. "Forensic Applications of DNA Fingerprinting." *Molecular Biotechnology*, vol. 1, no. 1, February 1994, pp. 13–27. This is an excellent review article that describes the technology of DNA typing and reviews some important forensic applications of the procedure.

Thompson, William C., F. Taroni, and C. G. G. Aitken. "How the Probability of a False Positive Affects the Value of DNA Evidence." *Journal of Forensic Sciences*, vol. 48, no. 1, January 2003, pp. 47–54. The authors review the causes of false positive results in DNA typing and argue that "ignorance of the true rate of error creates an important element of uncertainty about the value of DNA evidence." The article drew considerable discussion in later issues of the journal.

Thompson, William C. "A Sociological Perspective on the Science of Forensic DNA Testing." *University of California Davis Law Review*, vol. 30, no. 4, 1997, pp. 1,113–1,136. The author makes the observation that the results of DNA typing produced by forensic laboratories have a distinctively different "flavor" than evidence produced by laboratories unrelated to the forensic sciences. The former deal almost exclusively with the law enforcement community in one aspect or another and may feel inclined, therefore, to provide a slant to DNA results that the law enforcement community may feel helpful or useful.

Tracy, Paul E., and Vincent Morgan. "Big Brother and His Science Kit: DNA Databases for 21st Century Crime Control?" *Journal of Criminal Law & Criminology*, vol. 90, no. 2, Winter 2000, pp. 635–690. The authors provide an introduction to the technologies of DNA typing and discuss some of the very complex legal, social, and ethical issues posed by widespread use of these technologies in forensic science.

Tyler, Paul B. "Fundamental Misunderstandings about DNA Contamination: Does It Help or Hurt the Criminal Defendant?" *Beverly Hills Bar Association Journal*, vol. 31, Winter–Spring 1996, pp. 15–41. This article is an extended analysis of the effect of contamination in obtaining DNA evidence for criminal trials, written by a law clerk for the presiding judge in the O. J. Simpson case.

Valdivieso, Veronica. "DNA Warrants: A Panacea for Old, Cold Rape Cases?" *Georgetown Law Journal*, vol. 90, no. 4, April 2002, pp. 1,009+. The first part of this article provides a review of the current technology available for DNA profiling and the controversy over the admissibility and reliability of DNA fingerprints. The second part deals with the technical question of the constitutionality of warrants issued on the basis of DNA evidence.

Weedn, V. W., and R. K. Roby. "Forensic DNA Testing." *Archives of Pathology & Laboratory Medicine*. vol. 117, no. 5, May 1993, pp. 486–491. This is a good general review article dealing with the methodologies and forensic applications of DNA typing.

Williams, Robin, and Paul Johnson. "Inclusiveness, Effectiveness and Intrusiveness: Issues in the Developing Uses of DNA Profiling in Support of Criminal Investigations." *Journal of Law, Medicine & Ethics*, vol. 34, no 2, Summer 2006, pp. 234–247. The authors consider the social and ethical issues raised by the creation of large DNA databases accumulated during criminal investigations. They base much of their analysis on the history of DNA databases that have evolved in England and Wales over the past decades.

Word, Charlotte J. "The Future of DNA Testing and Law Enforcement." *Brooklyn Law Review*, vol. 67, no. 1, 2001, pp. 249–255. This article is a summary essay on the role of DNA typing in the future of forensic science, as part of a special issue on the topic of DNA typing in the journal.

Zagorski, Nick. "Profile of Alec J. Jeffreys." *Proceedings of the National Academy of Sciences*, vol. 103, no. 24, June 13, 2006, pp. 8918–8920. Zagorski reviews the discovery of restriction fragment length polymorphism (RFLP) analysis of DNA by Jeffreys and some of its earliest applications in forensic science and other fields.

Reports

Association of Chief Police Officers. *DNA Good Practice Manual.* 2nd ed., 2005. Available online. URL: http://www.forensic.gov.uk/forensic_t/inside/news/docs/DNA_Good.pdf#search=%22%22dna%20good%20practice%20manual%22%22. Accessed on July 28, 2007. Although designed for law enforcement officers in the United Kingdom, this document provides an excellent general background to the subject of DNA typing, its methodology, and its applications in forensic science.

Committee on DNA Forensic Science. National Research Council. *The Evaluation of Forensic DNA Evidence*. Washington, D.C.: National Academy Press, 1996. This report by a committee of the National Research Council follows up on an earlier report (1992) on DNA typing. It focuses narrowly on the principles of population genetics and statistics as they apply to DNA evidence. Major topics included in the book are "Genetic and Molecular Basis of DNA Typing," "Ensuring High Standards of Laboratory Performance," "Population Genetics," "Statistical Issues," and "DNA Evidence in the Legal System."

Committee on DNA Technology in Forensic Science. Board on Biology. Commission on Life Sciences. National Research Council. *DNA Technology in Forensic Science*. Washington, D.C.: National Academy Press, 1992. This report describes a study conducted by a committee of the National Research Council concerning the forensic applications of DNA typing. Chapters in the report include "DNA Typing: Technical Considerations," "DNA Typing: Statistical Basis for Interpretation," "Ensuring High Standards," "Forensic DNA Databanks and Privacy of Information," "Use of DNA Information in the Legal System," and "DNA Typing and Society."

Connors, Edward, Thomas Lundregan, Neal Miller, and Tom McEwen. *Convicted by Juries: Exonerated by Science*. Washington, D.C.: National Institute of Justice, June 1996. Available online. URL: http://www.ncjrs.

gov/pdffiles/dnaevid.pdf. The authors studied the cases of 28 individuals who had been convicted of crimes, served an average of seven years in prison, and then were released on the basis of DNA evidence.

Curran, Thomas. "Forensic DNA Analysis: Technology and Application. [Ottawa]: Library of Parliament, report no. BP443E, September 1997." This report provides an unusually good general overview of the technology and applications of DNA typing prepared for the Canadian parliament.

Easteal, Patricia Weiser, and Simon Easteal. "The Forensic Use of DNA Profiling." Trends and Issues in Crime and Criminal Justice, Paper number 26. Canberra: The Australian Institute of Criminology, November 1990. This report is a somewhat dated, but very thoughtful review of the social, legal, and ethical issues involved in DNA typing.

Gans, Jeremy, and Gregor Urbas. "DNA Identification in the Criminal Justice System." Trends and Issues in Crime and Criminal Justice, Paper number 226. Canberra: The Australian Institute of Criminology, May 2002. The report provides an excellent general overview of DNA typing that is understandable for almost anyone without a scientific or legal background.

Hammond, Holly A., and C. Thomas Caskey. "Automated DNA Typing: Method of the Future?" Washington, D.C.: National Institute of Justice, 1997. This report summarizes research conducted on DNA typing in an attempt to make the technology better adapted for use with samples collected at crime scenes.

Kreeger, Lisa R., and Danielle M. Weiss. *Forensic DNA Fundamentals for the Prosecutor: Be Not Afraid*. Alexandria, Va.: American Prosecutors Research Institute, 2003. Also available online. URL: http://www.ndaaapri.org/pdf/forensic_dna_fundamentals.pdf. This report is a publication in the American Prosecutors Research Institute's "Special Topics" series dealing with the technical aspects of DNA typing and legal issues involved in its admissibility in criminal cases.

———. *DNA Evidence Policy Considerations for the Prosecutor*. Alexandria, Va.: American Prosecutors Research Institute, 2004. This monograph summarizes key points made by the 200 participants of a conference on DNA typing sponsored by the institute in November 2003.

Lovrich, N. P., et al. *National Forensic DNA Study Report*. [Washington, D.C.:] U. S. Department of Justice, document number 203970, December 12, 2003. This document is the final report of a joint project conducted by researchers at Washington State University and Smith Alling Lane, P.S. on the magnitude of the DNA typing backlog, the reason for its existence, the capacity of existing laboratories to conduct DNA typing, and some ways in which the existing backlog can be handled.

National Commission on the Future of DNA Evidence. *The Future of Forensic DNA Testing*. Washington, D.C.: U.S. Department of Justice, Office of Justice Programs, 2000. This report summarizes the predictions of future DNA forensic use by the Research and Development Working Group. The major portion of the report is devoted to predictions for the role of DNA testing in 2002, 2005, and 2010, and a discussion of population and statistical issues involved in DNA testing.

———. *Using DNA to Solve Cold Cases.* Washington, D.C.: National Institute of Justice, 2002. The report considered a number of issues in the use of DNA typing to solve old, unsolved ("cold") criminal cases, taking into consideration advances in DNA technology, new laws, and statutes of limitation.

National Institute of Justice. *Report to the Attorney General on Delays in DNA Forensic Analysis.* Washington, D.C.: National Institute of Justice. U.S. Department of Justice, March 2003. In August 2001, Attorney General John Ashcroft directed the National Institute of Justice (NIJ) to study the reasons that DNA forensic analysis was not being used more efficiently in the investigation of criminal cases in the United States. This report contains the results of that study along with recommendations for changes that should be made to improve the efficacy of DNA typing in forensic science.

Steadman, Greg W. *Survey of DNA Crime Laboratories, 2001.* U.S. Department of Justice. Office of Justice Programs. Bureau of Justice Statistics Bulletin NCJ 191191, January 2002. This report describes a survey conducted in 2000 of 110 of the approximately 120 known public testing laboratories that conduct DNA typing. The study is the latest of its type available as of 2007 and complements a similar study conducted in 1998 (*Survey of DNA Crime Laboratories, 1998*, February 2000, report NCJ 179104).

Weedn, Victor Walter, and John W. Hicks. *The Unrealized Potential of DNA Testing.* U.S. Department of Justice. Office of Justice Programs. National Institute of Justice, June 1998. Also available online. URL: http://www.ncjrs.gov/pdffiles/170596.pdf#search=%22%22The%20Unrealized%20Potential%20of%20DNA%20Testing%22%22. A report from the National Institute of Justice acknowledges the important contributions that DNA testing has already made to law enforcement and criminal justice, but points out changes that should be made to permit the technology to reach its full potential. The most important steps are improved technology, additional funding, and the use of automated systems to permit networking of DNA typing information.

Web Documents

American Society of Law, Medicine, and Ethics. "DNA Fingerprinting and Civil Liberties—Project Homepage." Available online. URL: http://

www.aslme.org/dna_04/index.php. Accessed on March 27, 2007. This web page is a project funded by the Human Genome Research Institute of the National Institutes of Health (NIH) devoted to exploring the ethical, legal, and social issues related to the use of DNA typing. It contains complete accounts and reports of four workshops held in 2004 and 2005, as well as a number of special reports, important legal cases, and other reports on DNA typing relevant to the subject of this project.

Baden, Michael. "DNA Profiling." Available online. URL: http://www.kathyreichs.com/dnaprofiling.htm. Accessed on March 28, 2007. This web page is a well-illustrated general introduction to the technology involved in DNA typing.

Ballve, Marcelo. "DNA Fingerprinting Trend Threatens Genetic Privacy." Available online. URL: http://www.alternet.org/rights/19234/. Posted on July 14, 2004. The author expresses concern about the growing movement to obtain DNA "fingerprints" from people who are arrested for or suspected of crimes, even though they may not be convicted of or charged with such crimes.

BBC News. "DNA Profiling of Babies Rejected." Available online. URL: http://news.bbc.co.uk/1/hi/health/4396833.stm. Updated on March 31, 2005. The British government decides not to follow up on a proposal to do DNA typing of all newborn babies in the country (for possible health and medical reasons) because of legal, ethical, and social reasons.

Betsch, David F. "DNA Fingerprinting in Human Health and Society." Available online. URL: http://www.accessexcellence.org/RC/AB/BA/DNA_Fingerprinting_Basics.html. Accessed on March 28, 2007. This web page from the National Health Museum's Access Excellence program provides a brief introduction to the technology of DNA typing with links to other sources on the subject.

Biotechnology Online. "DNA Profiling." Available online. URL: http://www.biotechnologyonline.gov.au/human/dnaprofile.cfm. Accessed on March 25, 2007. This web page is an excellent interactive program in which the reader is allowed to go through the specific steps involved in analyzing DNA samples collected at the scene of a crime.

"Blackett Family DNA Activity 2." Available online. URL: http://www.biology.arizona.edu/human_bio/activities/blackett2/overview.html. Posted on October 27, 2000. This web page was developed by The Biology Project of the University of Arizona. It provides a complete and sophisticated introduction to the theory and practice of DNA typing using real DNA data provided by a DNA technician.

Brenner, Charles H. "Forensic Mathematics of DNA Matching." Available online. URL: http://dnaview.com/profile.htm. Accessed on March 28, 2007. This online tutorial provides instruction on the calculation of probabilities of DNA matches for advanced students of the subject.

Brinton, Kate, and Kim-An Lieberman. "Basics of DNA Fingerprinting." Available online. URL: http://protist.biology.washington.edu/fingerprint/dnaintro.html. Accessed on March 28, 2007. This web page provides a simple introduction to the technology of DNA typing with a glossary and suggested further readings.

Budowle, Bruce, Ranajit Chakraborty, George Carmody, and Keith L. Monson. "Source Attribution of a Forensic DNA Profile." *Forensic Science Communications*, vol. 2, no. 3, July 2000. Available online. URL: http://www.fbi.gov/hq/lab/fsc/backissu/july2000/source.htm#Abstract. Accessed on July 28, 2007. The authors advance a technical analysis of the statistical probabilities available from DNA typing and methods for interpreting the significance of those probabilities.

Burlingame, Laurie. "Forensic Use of DNA: Bibliography of Law Reviews and Journals." Available online. URL: http://www.aslme.org/dna_04/reports/burlingame.pdf. Accessed on March 27, 2007. This web page provides a summary of books and articles dealing with the legal, ethical, and social issues related to the development of DNA databases prepared for the American Society of Law, Medicine and Ethics conferences on DNA Forensics and Civil Liberties.

Casey, Denise. "What Can the New Gene Tests Tell Us?" *The Judges' Journal*, vol. 36, no. 3, Summer 1997. Available online. URL: http://www.ornl.gov/sci/techresources/Human_Genome/publicat/judges/judge.html. Accessed on July 28, 2007. The article provides a good general introduction to the technology of DNA typing and its applications in the courtroom, from a special journal issue on "Genetics in the Courtroom."

Cline, Erin. "DNA Fingerprinting—It's Everywhere!" Available online. URL: http://www.thetech.org/genetics/news.php?id=16. Accessed on March 28, 2007. Cline offers a nice general introduction to the use of DNA typing in forensic science with links to other articles in this series that deal with more technical aspects of DNA typing.

Colb, Sherry F. "A Federal Appeals Court Approves the DNA Profiling of Criminals: Are Innocent People Next?" Available online. URL: http://writ.news.findlaw.com/colb/20040908.html. Posted on September 8, 2004. Colb provides a commentary on the FindLaw web site that reports on a decision by the U.S. Court of Appeals for the Ninth Circuit that upheld the compulsory DNA profiling of convicted offenders through mandatory blood sampling. The author explores the consequences of this decision for individuals who are accused of or arrested for crimes, but not convicted of them, as well as for innocent people.

Crime Scene Investigation. "Free at Last!" Available online. URL: http://whyfiles.org/126dna_forensic/index.html. Posted on January 25, 2001. The web page contains a good general description of DNA typing that begins with the story of a prisoner who was exonerated of the crimes for which he was convicted on the basis of DNA evidence.

Crimtrac. "DNA." Available online. URL: http://www.crimtrac.gov.au/systems_projects_dna.html. Accessed on July 28, 2007. A project of the Australian government, this web page provides a good general introduction to the principles and methods of DNA typing, the Australian National Criminal Investigation DNA Database (NCIDD), and issues related to DNA profiling.

Defense Prisoner of War/Missing Personnel Office. "Deoxyribonucleic acid (DNA) Typing." Available online. URL: http://www.dtic.mil/dpmo/family_support_info/dnatyping.htm. Accessed on March 20, 2007. This web site explains the use of DNA typing in the identification of bodily remains of men and women killed or lost in earlier wars.

Division of Criminal Justice Services. State of New York. "The NYS DNA Databank and CODIS." Available online. URL: http://criminaljustice.state.ny.us/forensic/dnabrochure.htm. Accessed on March 28, 2007. This web page offers an excellent summary of the way the DNA databank in one state (New York) operates and summarizes the results that have been obtained as a result of the database and its affiliation with the FBI's CODIS system.

"DNA Analysis." Available online. URL: http://opbs.okstate.edu/~melcher/mg/MGW4/MG42.html. Last updated on October 22, 1998. This is an excellent web site that deals with the details of DNA typing technology taken from various parts of an extensive series of lecture notes for a course in Molecular Genetics, given by Ulrich Melcher at Oklahoma State University.

"DNA Fingerprinting." Available online. URL: http://www.biotech.iastate.edu/lab_protocols/DNA_Fingerprinting.html. Posted June 1994. This web page contains an experiment on DNA typing prepared by the Office of Biotechnology at Iowa State University.

"DNA Fingerprinting." Available online. URL: http://www.bergen.org/AAST/Projects/Gel/fingprint1.htm. Accessed on October 1, 2006. This web site offers a good general introduction to the history and technology of DNA typing with a discussion of some applications of the technology.

"DNA Testing: Introduction and Index." Available online. URL: http://www.vivo.colostate.edu/hbooks/genetics/medgen/dnatesting/. Last updated on March 18, 1996. This is a web page that provides a general overview of DNA typing including discussions, strengths, limitations and controversies about DNA typing; DNA polymorphisms; techniques of DNA typing; and applications of DNA typing.

European Initiative for Biotechnology Education, The. "Unit 2: DNA Profiling." Available online. URL: http://www.ipn.unikiel.de/eibe/ENGLISH/U2.HTM. Accessed on March 25, 2007. This web page contains a superb instructional unit on DNA typing with a complete and clear description of the theory involved, some practical issues involved in its use in forensic and other applications, and a laboratory exercise on typing.

Federal Bureau of Investigation. "CODIS: Combined DNA Index System." Available online. URL: http://www.fbi.gov/hq/lab/codis. Accessed on January 25, 2007. This web site is the home page for the FBI's Combined DNA Index System (CODIS) that contains in excess of four million profiles (as of 2007), of which about 160,000 are forensic profiles. The web site contains a description of the system, statistics, and recent news. A brochure outlining the program can also be accessed from this web page by clicking on the link "CODIS Brochure."

Gene Expression. Available online. URL:http://www.gnxp.com/. Accessed on March 25, 2007. This blog has an interesting exchange of viewpoints on DNA typing, especially the use of DNA databases.

Groleau, Rick. "Create a DNA Fingerprint." Available online. URL: http://www.pbs.org/wgbh/nova/sheppard/analyze.html. Last updated in November 2000. This web page allows readers to create and analyze a DNA fingerprint.

Human Genome Project Information. "DNA Forensics." Available online. URL: http://www.ornl.gov/sci/techresources/Human_Genome/elsi/forensics.shtml. Last modified June 14, 2006. This web page is a collection of basic information on DNA typing and its applications in forensic science. The site includes topics such as how forensic identification works; how DNA typing is done; some applications of DNA typing in forensic investigations; DNA forensic databases; ethical, legal, and social issues associated with DNA databanking; and potential benefits of DNA databanking. A number of links to other DNA typing sites is also provided.

Interpol. "DNA Profiling." Available online. URL: http://www.interpol.int/Public/Forensic/dna/default.asp. Accessed on March 20, 2007. This web page describes the structure and activities of Interpol, the world's largest international law enforcement agency.

Iowa Department of Public Safety. Division of Criminal Investigation. "The DCI DNA Profiling Section." Available online. URL: http://www.dps.state.ia.us/DCI/Crime_Lab/DNA/index.shtml. Accessed on July 28, 2007. This is an especially interesting web site because it provides a good insight on the instructions provided to law enforcement officers about the collection, testing, and interpretation of DNA profiles.

Jaksic, Vesna. "DNA Databases May Be Growing Too Quickly." Available online. URL: http://www.law.com/jsp/article.jsp?id=1169028144230. Accessed on January 27, 2007. Originally printed in the January 18, 2007, issue of *The National Law Journal*, this article reviews the rapid growth of

DNA databases throughout the states with some administrative and legal problems resulting from this change.

Jones, Philip B. C. "Arresting Developments in DNA Typing." Available online. URL: http://forensicevidence.com/site/Biol_Evid/BioEvid_dna_jones.html. Accessed on July 28, 2007. The authors provide a general introduction to the history of DNA typing, its current status in the United States, and some issues related to its use in forensic science.

KariSable.com. "Criminal Investigations, DNA & Forensic Science." Available online. URL: http://www.karisable.com/crdna1.htm. Accessed on March 28, 2007. This is a good web site with basic information about DNA typing and links to other web pages and organizations with additional and specialized information on the topic.

Kubow, Kristopher. "DNA Fingerprinting." *Illumin*, vol. 7, no. 1, November 1, 2001. Available online. URL: http://illumin.usc.edu/article.php?articleID=53&page=4. Accessed on July 28, 2007. Kubow provides an excellent general introduction to the technology of DNA typing and its applications in a variety of fields, including the forensic sciences.

Lawless, Jill. "DNA Fingerprinting Sparks Fresh Worries: Discoverer Says Genetic Databases Could Be Misused." Available online. URL: http://www.msnbc.msn.com/id/5944270/. Posted on September 8, 2004. The author discusses some of the ways in which DNA databases are being used with the potential for misuse that exists, with a commentary by Alec Jeffreys, discoverer of the RFLP DNA typing procedure.

Lewis, Simon W. "DNA Typing." Available online. URL: http://caligula.bcs.deakin.edu.au/bcs_courses/forensic/Chemical%20Detective/DNA_Type.htm. Last updated on June 13, 2005. This is a clear and well-written introduction to the general principles of DNA typing.

Lonsway, Kimberly A. "DNA Evidence and Issues." A module prepared in conjunction with "Successfully Investigating Acquaintance Sexual Assault: A National Training Manual for Law Enforcement." Available online. URL: http://www.denverda.org/DNA_Documents/DNA%20Evidence%20&%20Issues.pdf. Accessed on March 28, 2007. The author provides an extended discussion of the way in which DNA typing can be used in the investigation of rape crimes.

Marion Koshland Museum of the National Academy of Sciences. "Putting DNA to Work." Available online. URL: http://www.koshlandsciencemuseum.org/exhibitdna/crim01.jsp. Accessed on March 20, 2007. This web page includes an instructional unit on DNA typing, suggested teaching activities, links to related web pages, and additional reading resources.

Martin, Carolyn Napier. "DNA Fingerprinting: You Be the Judge!" Available online. URL: http://www.woodrow.org/teachers/bi/1992/DNA_printing.html. Accessed on March 28, 2007. This exercise is designed for beginning biology students. It provides them with the opportunity to analyze DNA typing data and reach a conclusion as to the information those data provide in a criminal case.

Mayo, Ellen, and Anthony Bertino. "Where's the CAT? A DNA Profiling Simulation." Available online. URL: http://www.accessexcellence.org/AE/AEC/AEF/1995/mayo_dna.html. Accessed on March 25, 2007. This is an exercise for students in grade 7 to adult that simulates the laboratory steps involved in the production of a DNA profile.

Medical News Today. "First Test of Rapid DNA Analysis Pioneered by Washington State and Orchid Cellmark Identifies Alleged Child Rapist Within Just Days." Available online. URL: http://www.medicalnewstoday.com/medicalnews.php?newsid=65063. Posted on March 13, 2007. This report describes a new technological development with which DNA typing can be completed within a matter of about a week compared to the usual time of six months or more.

Meeker-O'Connell, Ann. "How DNA Evidence Works." How Stuff Works. Available online. URL: http://science.howstuffworks.com/dnaevidence.htm. Accessed on August 21, 2006. This web page offers an easy-to-understand description of DNA typing technology with a review of recent advances in the field and a discussion of applications of the procedure.

Moskowitz, Ellen. "Forensic Use of DNA: Summary of Selected Law Review and Law Journal Articles." Available online. URL: http://www.aslme.org/dna_04/reports/moskowitz.pdf. Accessed on August 21, 2006. This is an excellent annotated bibliography of legal articles on DNA typing ranging from 1993 to 2003.

Myers, Richard. "DNA Fingerprinting for High School Biology." Available online. URL: http://www.accessexcellence.org/AE/AEC/AEF/1996/myers_dna.html. Accessed on March 28, 2007. This laboratory experiment on DNA typing, designed for high school students, is offered as part of the National Museum of Health's Access Excellence web page.

National Commission on the Future of DNA Evidence. *What Every Law Enforcement Officer Should Know about DNA Evidence*. Available online. URL: http://www.ncjrs.gov/pdffiles1/nij/bc000614.pdf. Accessed on July 28, 2007. This brief booklet outlines essential information about DNA typing and its use in criminal investigations.

National Conference of State Legislatures. "DNA & Crime." Available online. URL: http://www.ncsl.org/programs/health/genetics/dna.htm. Accessed on March 28, 2007. This collection of print publications, Internet sites, and other resources deals with the use of DNA evidence in the criminal justice system, including issues such as the admissibility of DNA evidence, policies governing the maintenance of DNA databanks, and offenses qualifying for DNA collection.

National Conference of State Legislatures. "DNA 2003." Available online. URL: http://www.ncsl.org/programs/health/genetics/dna2003.htm. Accessed on March 28, 2007. This summary of legislation passed in the 50 states on the forensic uses of DNA was a one-time study that was not repeated in later years.

National Criminal Justice Reference System. "In the Spotlight." Available online. URL: http://www.ncjrs.gov/spotlight/forensic/legislation.html. Accessed on August 21, 2006. This is a summary of online federal and state legislation, important court decisions, and federal rules of evidence relating to DNA typing.

National Institute of Forensic Science Australia. "DNA Profiling." Available online. URL: http://www.nifs.com.au/F_S_A/FSA_frame.html?DNA_Profiling.asp&1. Accessed on March 25, 2007. This general overview deals with the technology and applications in forensic science of DNA typing with a glossary and links to other resources.

Newton, Giles. "Discovering DNA Fingerprinting." Available online. URL: http://genome.wellcome.ac.uk/doc_wtd020877.html. Accessed on August 21, 2006. Newton reviews the discovery of DNA typing and some early cases in which it was used.

Newton's Apple. "DNA Fingerprinting." Available online. URL: http://www.reachoutmichigan.org/funexperiments/agesubject/lessons/newton/dna.html. Accessed on March 28, 2007. This episode of the *Newton's Apple* television program provides a brief general introduction to DNA typing with instructions for carrying out a simple experiment in chromatography.

Nihiser, Michele L. "The Advances of DNA Technology and Its Effects on The Criminal Justice System." Available online. URL: http://dscholarship.lib.fsu.edu/undergrad/201/. Accessed on July 28, 2007. This paper, presented as an undergraduate honors thesis at Florida State University, provides a thorough and well-written review of the development of DNA typing technology and its applications in forensic science.

O'Connor, Thomas R. "DNA Typing and Identification." Available online. URL: http://faculty.ncwc.edu/TOConnor/425/425lect15.htm. Updated February 6, 2006. This is a very complete, well-written review of DNA typing technology developed for a course in criminal justice at Austin Peay State University in Fort Campbell, Kentucky.

Pickrell, John. "Supersensitive Profiling Deciphers Wisps of DNA." *New Scientist*, vol. 16, no. 12, October 4, 2006. Available online. URL: http://www.newscientist.com/article.ns?id=dn10225&feedId=onlinenews_rss20. Accessed on July 28, 2007. The article reports on a new method for conducting DNA tests that may increase crime detection rates by up to 15 percent.

Porter, Sandra G. "A DNA Fingerprinting Exercise for Any Type of Class." Available online. URL: http://www.geospiza.com/education/docs/DNA_fingerprinting.pdf. Accessed on August 21, 2006. This report on a Seattle Central Community College (SCCC) unit on DNA typing contains a nice general introduction to the technology and applications of DNA typing, as well as a description of a DNA typing experiment designed for the SCCC class.

President's DNA Initiative. *Advancing Justice through DNA Technology*. Available online. URL: http://www.dna.gov/info/. Accessed on July 28, 2007. The President's DNA Initiative originated in an August 2001 order by then attorney general John Ashcroft to the National Institute for Justice to conduct a study on the delays that occur in the use of DNA evidence in the criminal justice and to recommend changes that would reduce or eliminate those delays. Based on the results of that study, President George W. Bush announced the President's DNA Initiative on March 11, 2003. That initiative called for a five-year $1 billion program to increase funding, training, and assistance for DNA technology at the federal, state, and local levels. This report contains the details of that initiative.

———. "Forensic DNA Databases." Available online. URL: http://www.dna.gov/uses/database. Accessed on January 27, 2007. This general overview of DNA databases maintained by the U.S. federal government also includes suggestions for additional research in outside sources.

———. *Principles of Forensic DNA for Officers of the Court*. Available online. URL: http://www.dna.gov/training/#online. This document is an interactive resource for prosecutors, defense attorneys, and judges on the principles of DNA typing and their application in forensic science. Registration for the online course is free.

Ramsland, Katherine. *The DNA Revolution* (ebook). Available online. URL: http://www.crimelibrary.com/criminal_mind/forensics/dna/1.html. Accessed on March 28, 2007. This electronic book in the Crime Library series provides some historical background on DNA typing, the technology involved, its applications in the forensic sciences, and some issue raised by DNA typing.

"Restriction Fragment Length Polymorphisms (RFLPs)." Available online. URL: http://users.rcn.com/jkimball.ma.ultranet/BiologyPages/R/RFLPs.html. Accessed on March 28, 2007. This web page contains a very technical description of the methods by which RFLP technology is carried out.

Riley, Donald E. "DNA Testing: An Introduction for Non-Scientists; An Illustrated Explanation." *Scientific Testimony, an Online Journal*. Available online. URL: http://www.scientific.org/tutorials/articles/riley/riley.html. Posted on April 6, 2005. This web site offers a simplified illustrated introduction to the technology of DNA typing for those who have "limited backgrounds in biological sciences."

Rosner, Dalya, and Chris Smith. "How Does Genetic Fingerprinting Work?" The Naked Scientists Guest Columnists. Available online. URL: http://www.thenakedscientists.com/html/columnists/dalyacolumn8.htm. This web page offers a general introduction to the technology and applications of DNA typing with links to a number of related articles on the Naked Scientists web site dealing with topics such as the basics of DNA fingerprinting, how to make a DNA fingerprint, DNA fingerprinting using variable numbers of tandem repeats, the history of DNA, questions and answers about DNA fingerprinting, DNA transposons, and an interview with Alec Jeffreys, discoverer of DNA typing.

Royal Chemical Society. "DNA Profiling." Available online. URL: http://www.chemsoc.org/ExemplarChem/entries/2003/hull_barry/AG%20DNA%20Profiling.htm#PCR. Accessed on March 25, 2007. This web page provides a succinct introduction to the technical background on which DNA typing is based.

Russo, Juliana C. "Fourth Amendment Challenges to DNA Databanks in State Courts." Available online. URL: http://www.aslme.org/dna_04/reports/russo_update.pdf. Accessed on March 25, 2007. This report, prepared for the American Society of Law, Medicine, and Ethics, summarizes the status of cases that have been raised in the states about the creation and implementation of DNA databases.

Science Buddies. "Who Done It?" Available online. URL: http://www.sciencebuddies.org/mentoring/project_ideas/BioChem_p009.shtml?from=Home. Updated on July 12, 2006. This science project on DNA typing provides a relatively simple introduction and instructions for carrying out a DNA typing experiment.

Science Odyssey, A. "DNA 'Fingerprinting.'" PBS Resources for Educators. Available online. URL: http://www.pbs.org/wgbh/aso/resources/guide/earthact3index.html. Accessed on March 28, 2007. This activity for high school level students includes a good exercise on using DNA typing to determine parentage.

University of Michigan. "DNA Fingerprinting, Genetics and Crime: DNA Testing and the Courtroom." Available online. URL: http://www.fathom.com/course/21701758/index.html. Accessed on March 20, 2007. This web page, prepared as part of the university's Fathom seminar series, offers a sophisticated review of the technology of DNA typing and its applications in forensic science, with special attention to issues raised by the technology.

White, Ray. "A Brief History of Forensic DNA Typing." Available online. URL: http://www.cstl.nist.gov/div831/strbase/ppt/intro.pdf. Accessed on

October 10, 2006. This powerpoint presentation reviews the history of DNA fingerprinting, the basic technology involved in the procedure, and some important applications in the forensic sciences.

Wittmeyer, Jacqui. "Can DNA Demand a Verdict?" Available online. URL: http://learn.genetics.utah.edu/features/forensics/. Accessed on March 25, 2007. The author provides a general introduction to DNA typing and its applications in forensic science. The web page was developed by the Genetic Science Learning Center at the University of Utah.

Winickoff, David. "The Constitutionality of Forensic DNA Databanks: 4th Amendment Issues." Available online. URL: http://www.aslme.org/dna_04/reports/winickoff_update.pdf. Updated on June 30, 2005. This paper on the legal aspects of DNA typing was prepared for a 2004 workshop sponsored by the American Society of Law, Medicine, and Ethics.

Zedlewski, Edwin, and Mary B. Murphy. "DNA Analysis for 'Minor' Crimes: A Major Benefit for Law Enforcement." *NIJ Journal*, no. 253, January 2006. Available online. URL: http://www.ojp.usdoj.gov/nij/journals/253/dna_analysis.html. Accessed on July 28, 2007. Although DNA testing is usually associated with murder cases and other violent crimes, the authors point out that it can be used in the investigation of many less serious offenses.

CHAPTER 8

ORGANIZATIONS AND AGENCIES

This chapter contains information on agencies, associations, organizations, and other groups whose primary or exclusive focus involves some aspect of fingerprint analysis, ballistic fingerprinting, DNA typing, or polygraph testing. (There are no organizations whose interest lies in the Bertillonage form of anthropometry.) The list of organizations is divided into two general categories: Governmental Organizations and Professional Organizations.

GOVERNMENTAL ORGANIZATIONS

Armed Forces DNA Identification Laboratory (AFDIL)
URL: http://www.afip.org/Departments/oafme/dna/
c/o Armed Forces Institute of Pathology
6825 16th Street, N.W.
Washington, DC 20306-6000

The mission of the Armed Forces DNA Identification Laboratory (AFDIL) is twofold: (1) "to provide worldwide scientific consultation, research, and education services in the field of forensic DNA analysis to the Department of Defense (DoD) and other agencies," and (2) "to provide DNA reference specimen collection, accession, and storage of United States military and other authorized personnel." The major task of the AFDIL is to use DNA technology to identify members of the armed services who have been killed or lost in battles and who would or have otherwise remained unidentified.

Bureau of Alcohol, Tobacco, Firearms and Explosives (ATF)
U.S. Department of the Treasury
URL: http://www.atf.treas.gov/
E-mail: ATFMail@atf.gov
Office of Public and Governmental Affairs
650 Massachusetts Avenue, N.W.
Room 8290
Washington, DC 20226

The Bureau of Alcohol, Tobacco, and Firearms (ATF) was created by

Treasury Department Order No. 221 on July 1, 1972, which transferred from the Internal Revenue Service (IRS) responsibility for all federal laws and regulations dealing with alcohol, tobacco, firearms, and explosives. The bureau's responsibilities have been expanded on later occasions to include control of interstate trafficking in contraband cigarettes (1978) and supervision of all commercial arson investigations in the United States (1982). Some of the agency's many responsibilities in connection with firearms include control of illegal trafficking, possession, and use of firearms; issuance of firearm licenses; and conduct of inspections of firearm dealers for compliance with federal regulations.

Department of Defense Academy for Credibility Assessment (DoDPI)
URL: http://www.dodpi.army.mil
Phone: (803) 751-9100
7540 Pickens Avenue
Fort Jackson, SC 29207

The U.S. Army Polygraph School was created in 1951 as a unit of the Provost Marshal General School at Fort Gordon, Georgia, and transferred to Fort McClellan, Alabama, in 1975. It was renamed the Department of Defense Polygraph Institute (DoDPI) in 1986 and given its current name on January 25, 2007. The academy has retained its acronym of DoDPI for many purposes. The school has a number of responsibilities related to polygraph use, including the training of all polygraph operators employed by the federal government, offering ongoing classes in polygraph use, and conducting research on new polygraph instruments and techniques. In the most recent year for which data are available, fiscal year 2002, DoDPI conducted 11,566 polygraph examinations, the largest number of which (8,512) were for counterintelligence purposes.

Federal Bureau of Investigation (FBI)
URL: http://www.fbi.gov
Phone: (202) 324-3000
J. Edgar Hoover Building
935 Pennsylvania Avenue, NW
Washington, DC 20535-0001

The Federal Bureau of Investigation (FBI) was established in 1908 by Attorney General Charles Bonaparte as a means of professionalizing law enforcement at the federal level in the United States. Today, the FBI is still responsible for investigating all violations of federal law except for those that have been specifically assigned to other agencies by way of legislation. The bureau's Criminal Justice Information Services Division (CJIS) maintains the world's largest collection of fingerprints as part of its National Repository of Criminal History Records and Criminal History Data (NRCHRCHD) program, roughly half of which are of criminals and half, non-criminals.

FBI National Academy Associates, Inc. (FBINAA)
URL: http://www.fbinaa.org/
E-mail: info@fbinaa.org

Phone: (703) 632-1990
National Executive Office
FBI Academy
Quantico, VA 22135

The FBI National Academy Associates, Inc. (FBINAA) was founded in 1935 to provide advanced training and the promotion of cooperation among law enforcement officers around the world. More than 36,000 men and women have graduated from the academy, and about half of those graduates have accepted the opportunity to become associates of the academy. Associates receive special benefits, such as a subscription to the academy's official publication, *The Associate*, as well as the opportunity to interact with other associates and have access to a variety of FBINAA resources.

Interpol
URL: http://www.interpol.int/
General Secretariat
200, quai Charles de Gaulle
69006 Lyon
France

Interpol is an international law enforcement agency created in 1923 and currently consisting of 186 nation members. The agency consists of five parts: a general assembly, a governing body that meets annually and consists of delegates from each member nation; the executive committee, a 13-member group elected by the general assembly; the general secretariat, located in Lyon, France, in charge of day-to-day operations with six regional offices in Argentina, Côte d'Ivoire, El Salvador, Kenya, Thailand, and Zimbabwe; national central bureaus, maintained by each member country, serving as a contact point for the general secretariat; and advisers, experts in certain specific areas of forensic science appointed by the executive committee and confirmed by the general assembly. Interpol's three core functions are to maintain a worldwide communication system through which information about crime and criminals can be shared, maintenance of databases in areas such as fingerprints and DNA profiles, and support services for national law enforcement agencies in areas such as drugs and organized crime, public safety and terrorism, and illegal trafficking in human beings and goods.

National Center for Forensic Science (NCFS)
URL: http://www.ncfs.org/home.html
Email: natlctr@mail.ucf.edu
Phone: (407) 823-6469
University of Central Florida
12354 Research Parkway
P. O. Box 162367
Orlando, FL 32816-2367

The National Center for Forensic Science (NCFS) is a program of the National Institute of Justice hosted by the University of Central Florida that offers a number of courses in forensic science, including advanced fire debris analysis, basic fire debris analysis, AccessData Windows Forensics, Gray Hat Research: Enterprise Network Forensics and Threat Profiling, AccessData Advance Internet

Forensics, and biological evidence. The mission of NCFS is to provide "research, education, training, tools and technology to meet the current and future needs of the forensic science, investigative and criminal justice communities."

National Center for Health Statistics (NCHS)
URL: http://www.cdc.gov/nchs/
E-mail: nchsquery@cdc.gov
Phone: (866) 441NCHS (6247)
3311 Toledo Road
Hyattsville, MD 20782

The National Center for Health Statistics (NCHS) is an agency of the National Institutes of Health (NIH) with the primary responsibility for collecting, evaluating, and disseminating data on health issues in the United States. Some uses of the NCHS data are documenting the health status of the U.S. population as a whole and of certain subgroups; identifying disparities in health status and use of health care among various racial, ethnic, socioeconomic, regional, and other categories; monitoring health status and health care delivery systems; identifying health problems; supporting biomedical and health sciences research; evaluating the impact of health policies and programs; and providing information for making changes in health policy and programs. NCHS is the repository of large amounts of anthropometric data that have been collected on populations in the United States and other parts of the world.

National Clearinghouse for Science, Technology and the Law (NCSTL)
URL: http://www.ncstl.org/
Phone: (727) 562-7316
Stetson University College of Law
1401 61st Street South
Gulfport, FL 33707

The National Clearinghouse for Science, Technology and the Law (NCSTL) was established in 2003 by a grant from the National Institute of Justice, Office of Justice Programs, U.S. Department of Justice for the purpose of providing judges, attorneys, scientists, and law enforcement officers with the information they need to understand and deal with legal problems that have a significant scientific and/or technological component. Among the services offered by NCSTL are "a searchable database of legal, forensic, and technology resources; a reference collection of law, science, and technology material; partnerships with law schools, professional associations, and federal and state agencies; national conferences on science, technology, and the law; community acceptance panels; training modules and primers with an emphasis on distance education; and training for defense counsel who are handling cases involving biological evidence on the applications and limitations of DNA evidence as stated in the President's DNA Initiative." Plans for additional services include additional distance education programs and expanded partnerships with law schools, professional organizations, and federal and state law enforcement agencies.

National Crime Information Center (NCIC)
URL: http://www.fas.org/irp/agency/doj/fbi/is/ncic.htm
Phone: (304) 625-2000
1000 Custer Hollow Road
Clarksburg, WV 26306

The National Crime Information Center (NCIC) was established in 1973 to provide a central clearing house for information on a wide variety of criminals and crimes. Today the center has information on topics such as stolen vehicles, boats, and articles; counterfeited bills and securities; wanted persons; foreign fugitives; delinquent children and adolescents; and missing persons. Information on all of these categories is available to qualified agencies and individuals in the law enforcement profession by contacting NCIC.

National Criminal Justice Reference Service (NCJRS)
URL: http://www.ncjrs.gov/
Phone: (800) 851-3420
P.O. Box 6000
Rockville, MD 20849-6000

The National Criminal Justice Reference Service (NCJRS) is a service sponsored by various agencies within the U.S. Department of Justice and the Office of National Drug Control Policy of the Executive Office of the President that offers a number of services free of charge to anyone interested in forensic issues. These services include reference and referral services on questions about crime and law enforcement research, policy, and practice; information about new publications, grants and funding opportunities, and other news and announcements; access to JUSTINFO, a biweekly electronic newsletter with e-mail notifications about training sessions, conferences, funding opportunities, and other matters; access to a host of articles, books, reports, and other publications in the field of law enforcement and forensic science; access to *The Justice Resource Update*, a quarterly publication about activities of NCJRS partners; and information about meetings and conferences on forensic issues. NCJRS maintains one of the largest criminal justice holdings in the world with more than 190,000 publications, reports, articles, and audiovisual products from the United States and other nations.

National Forensic Science Technology Center (NFSTC)
URL: http://www.nfstc.org/index.htm
E-mail: info@nfstc.org
Phone: (727) 549-6067
7881 114th Avenue North
Largo, FL 33773

The National Forensic Science Technology Center (NFSTC) was established in 1995 as a non-profit corporation by the American Society of Crime Laboratory Directors (ASCLD) for the purpose of providing training programs and quality support systems for forensic science programs throughout the

United States. NFSTC works in cooperation with the Office of Science and Technology in the National Institute of Justice to provide forensic products and services at no cost to all publicly funded crime laboratories in the United States. Some programs developed by NFSTC include: the creation of a training program for new and experience firearms examiners, in cooperation with the Association of Firearms and Tool Marks Examiners and the California Forensic Science Institute; the development of a DNA audit program for forensic laboratories that provide DNA typing services; and a training program for officers of the court on DNA typing procedures and interpretation.

National Institute of Justice (NIJ)
URL: http://www.ojp.usdoj.gov/nij/
Phone: (202) 307–2942
810 Seventh Street, NW
Washington, DC 20531

The National Institute of Justice (NIJ) is the research, development, and evaluation agency of the U.S. Department of Justice. It is responsible for conducting research on crime control and justice issues and provides objective, independent, evidence-based knowledge and tools to deal with crime and justice issues, particularly at the state and local levels. Some current major programs of the institute are the Violence against Women and Family Violence Research and Evaluation Program, Data Resources Program, National Criminal Justice Reference Service, and The President's DNA Initiative.

National Institute of Standards and Technology (NIST)
Information Access Division (IAD)
Image Group
URL: http://www.itl.nist.gov/iad/894.03/fing/fing.html
E-mail: inquiries@nist.gov
Phone: (301) 975-6478
100 Bureau Drive, Stop 8940
Gaithersburg, MD 208998940

The Image Group is the section within the National Institute of Standards and Technology's Information Access Division (IAD) responsible for research on fingerprinting. The general mission of the IAD it to "provide measurements and standards to advance technologies dealing with access to multimedia and other complex information." The Image Group has conducted a number of studies on various scientific aspects of fingerprint analysis, with special emphasis on the development of computerized and other sophisticated methods for collecting and analyzing fingerprint impressions.

National Integrated Ballistic Information Network (NIBIN)
Bureau of Alcohol, Tobacco, Firearms, and Explosives
Department of the Treasury
URL: http://www.nibin.gov/
E-mail: atfnibin@atf.gov
Phone: (202) 927-5660
650 Massachusetts Avenue, NW
Washington, DC 20226

The National Integrated Ballistic Information Network (NIBIN) was established by the Bureau of Alcohol, Tobacco and Firearms in 1997 to bring together ballistics databases from a number of sources into a single, unified network through which information from all sources can be shared with all participants. The network makes use of the ATF's Integrated Ballistic Identification System (IBIS) equipment, which allows forensic investigators to access digital images of the markings made by a firearm on bullets and cartridge casings. These images provide an automated initial comparison, which allows examiners to decide whether a sufficient match exists to permit more detailed analysis.

PROFESSIONAL ORGANIZATIONS

Academy of Criminal Justice Sciences (ACJS)
URL: http://www.acjs.org/
Phone: (301) 446-6300
P.O. Box 960
Greenbelt, MD 20768-0960

The Academy of Criminal Justice Sciences (ACJS) was established in 1963 for the purpose of promoting professional and scholarly activities in the field of criminal justice. It works to improve criminal justice education and to promote research and policy analysis in the field of criminal justice. The academy consists of scholars who are interested in research in criminal justice, professionals from all sectors of the criminal justice system, and students who are training to become members of the criminal justice profession.

American Academy of Forensic Sciences (AAFS)
URL: http://www.aafs.org/
Phone: (719) 636-1100
410 North 21st Street
Colorado Springs, CO 80904

The American Academy of Forensic Sciences (AAFS) was founded in 1948 and is dedicated "to the promotion of education and the elevation of accuracy, precision, and specificity in the forensic sciences." The organization has about 6,000 members from the fields of medicine, law, dentistry, toxicology, physical anthropology, document examination, psychiatry, physics, engineering, criminalistics, and education. It is divided into 10 specialty areas, including criminalistics, engineering sciences, jurisprudence, odontology, pathology/biology, physical anthropology, psychiatry/behavioral sciences, questioned documents, and toxicology.

American Association of Police Polygraphists, Inc. (AAPP)
URL: http://www.policepolygraph.org
Phone: (888) 743-5479
Waynesville, OH 45068

The American Association of Police Polygraphists, Inc. (AAPP) is an association of polygraph operators who work in some aspect of law enforcement for federal, state, local, or other jurisdictions. In addition to active members who fall into this category, the association also has honorary, affiliate, and life memberships for individuals interested in the organization's goals and activities but who do not qualify for active membership. The association sponsors annual seminars dealing with recent developments in the field.

American Board of Criminalistics (ABC)
URL: http://www.criminalistics.com/
E-mail: abcreg@dwave.net
Phone: (715) 845-3684
P.O. Box 1123
Wausau, WI 54402-1123
The American Board of Criminalistics (ABC) was established in 1989 to provide a national certification program for professionals in the field of the forensic sciences. The board offers three levels of certification: diplomate, fellow, and technical specialist. The latter two certificates are awarded to individuals who are employed in some field of forensic science, have demonstrated competence in that field, and, in the case of the fellow certificate, have passed specialized examinations in various fields of forensic science, while the diplomate certificate is awarded to anyone who meets these criteria and also passes a General Knowledge Examination developed by the board.

American Board of Forensic Psychology (ABFP)
URL: http://www.abpp.org
E-mail: office@abpp.org
Phone: (800) 255-7792
300 Drayton Street
3rd Floor
Savannah, GA 31401
The American Board of Forensic Psychology (ABFP) is one of 13 specialty boards that make up the American Board of Professional Psychology (ABBP). ABBP was organized to offer certification of specialization in a variety of fields of psychology, such as cognitive and behavioral psychology, clinical psychology, clinical child and adolescent psychology, clinical health psychology, and clinical neuropsychology, as well as forensic psychology. The board offers oral and written examinations that lead to special certificates in each of these fields, certificates that are generally recognized by hospitals, health systems, and other organizations.

American College of Forensic Examiners Institute of Forensic Science (ACFEI)
URL: http://www.acfei.com/
Phone: (800) 423-9737
2750 East Sunshine Street
Springfield, MO 65804
The American College of Forensic Examiners Institute of Forensic Science (ACFEI) is a membership organization consisting of forensic examiners—individuals who carry out tests needed to form expert opinions on some matter related to a criminal investigation. ACFEI's mission is to promote the dissemi-

nation of forensic information and provide the training needed to help forensic examiners remain up to date on current developments in the field. The association provides training courses, lectures, and other educational programs through which individuals can earn certification in a variety of fields, including homeland security, forensic consulting, medical investigation, forensic accounting, and forensic nursing.

American Polygraph Association (APA)
URL: http://www.polygraph.org
Email: manager@polygraph.org
Phone: (800) APA-8037
P.O. Box 8037
Chattanooga, TN 37414-0037
Established in 1966, the American Polygraph Association (APA) now consists of more than 3,200 professional polygraph analysts employed by private businesses; law enforcement agencies; and other branches of federal, state, and local government. The organization establishes standards for the education of polygraphers and for techniques and instruments used in the profession. It also provides continuing education and training for members of the profession and inspects schools and colleges offering courses and degrees in polygraphy to make sure that professional standards are maintained.

American Prosecutors Research Institute (APRI)
URL: http://www.ndaaapri.org/apri/index.html
Phone: (703) 549-9222
99 Canal Center Plaza
Suite 510
Alexandria, VA 22314
The American Prosecutors Research Institute (APRI) was created in 1984 by the National District Attorneys Association to act as its research and program development arm. Some of the services provided by APRI to prosecuting attorneys include case law information, current information on the status of relevant legislation, assistance in trial preparation, access to experts and presenters, assistance with policy development, material on specific topics, training in all states of prosecutorial work, information on relevant technologies, background on the effectiveness of various different sentencing alternatives, information on promising practices, and assistance with grant development.

American Society of Crime Laboratory Directors (ASCLD)
URL: http://www.ascld.org
Phone: (919) 773-2044
139K Technology Drive
Garner, NC 27529
The American Society of Crime Laboratory Directors (ASCLD) was founded in 1974 by a group of directors of crime laboratories throughout the United States. Members come from a wide range of academic disciplines, including biology, chemistry, document examination, physics, toxicology, education, and law enforcement. The organization's purpose is "to foster professional interests, assist the development of laboratory management principles

and techniques; acquire, preserve and disseminate forensic based information; maintain and improve communications among crime laboratory directors; and to promote, encourage and maintain the highest standards of practice in the field."

Association of Firearm and Tool Mark Examiners (AFTE)
URL: http://www.afte.org

The Association of Firearm and Tool Mark Examiners (AFTE) was founded in Chicago in 1969 by a group of about three dozen law enforcement and civilian specialists who had been meeting informally to discuss problems of common interest for a number of years. The original purpose of the association was to provide a forum for "the presentation of scientific and technical papers, descriptions of new techniques and procedures, review of instrumentation and the solution of common problems encountered in these scientific fields [firearm and tool mark identification]." AFTE carries out a number of activities, including support of research in the area of firearm and tool mark identification, scholarship support for students interested in majoring in this field, an annual training seminar in firearm and tool mark identification techniques, and publication of the *AFTE Journal.*

Association of Forensic DNA Analysts and Administrators (AFDAA)
URL: http://www.afdaa.org/

The Association of Forensic DNA Analysts and Administrators (AFDAA) is a nonprofit organization of individuals involved in forensic and legal applications of DNA typing. AFDAA currently has more than 200 members from over 75 agencies and companies in 25 states. The primary goals of the organization are to help members stay up to date on current methods, techniques, and procedures used in DNA typing; to disseminate information on research and development of new techniques in the field; to provide a forum for discussions on legislative issues concerning DNA analysis; to provide an avenue for networking with other DNA crime laboratories and personnel; to offer formal training and lectures on DNA typing; and to share and troubleshoot forensic DNA data and/or issues.

ASTM International
Committee E52 on Forensic Psychophysiology
URL: http://www.astm.org
Phone: (610) 832-9804
100 Barr Harbor Drive
PO Box C700
West Conshohocken, PA 19428-2959

Committee E52 of ASTM was formed in 1998 for the purpose of developing standards for the use of a variety of technologies and procedures used in the forensic sciences—polygraph testing included. The committee consists of about 80 members who meet twice a year to discuss and develop standards. Thus far, 15 standards in the field have been published.

The Biometric Consortium
URL: http://www.biometrics.org/
E-mail: Info@biometrics.org

The Biometric Consortium is concerned with research, development, testing, evaluation, and application of biometric-based methods for personal identification and verification, including technologies such as fingerprinting, hand geometry, handwriting, retinal and iris scans, voice prints, and facial characteristics. The consortium's primary activity is an annual biometrics conference held every fall. The organization works in close cooperation with the U.S. Department of Defense Biometrics Management Office and the National Science and Technology Council's Subcommittee on Biometrics to conduct research and develop standards of identification and recognition.

British Academy of Forensic Sciences (BAFS)
URL: http://www.bafs.org.uk
E-mail: Bafs@bafs.org.uk
Phone: 44 020 7837 0069
104 Barnsbury Road
Islington
London N1 0ES
United Kingdom

The British Academy of Forensic Sciences (BAFS) was formed in 1960 to promote the study and improve the practice of forensic science and medicine, to hold meetings and publish materials related to forensic science, and to promote the development of skills of those working in the fields of forensic science and forensic medicine. BAFS achieves these objectives by (1) promoting better cooperation between lawyers and expert witnesses, (2) providing expertise in the resolution of legal conflicts, and (3) working toward the solution of national and international problems in forensic science. The organization's official journal is *Medical Science and the Law*, which is published quarterly.

Canadian Identification Society (CIS)
URL: http://www.cissci.ca/
E-mail: admin@cis-sci.ca
19 Candow Crescent
Stittsville, ON K2S 1K7
Canada

The Canadian Identification Society (CIS) was created in 1977 after a somewhat lengthy gestation period that began about two decades earlier. The purpose of the organization is to ensure common and adequate standards among identification experts throughout Canada. The organization offers training programs and sponsors an annual convention.

Canadian Society of Forensic Science (CSFS)
La Société Canadienne des Sciences Judiciaires
URL: http://www.csfs.ca/index.htm
E-mail: csfs@bellnet.ca
Phone: (613) 7380001
3332 McCarthy Road
P.O. Box 37040
Ottawa, Ontario, K1V 0W0
Canada

The Canadian Society of Forensic Science (CSFS) was founded in 1953 during an informal meeting of 17 people involved in forensic science in Ottawa. The organization has grown to more than 450 members in the fields of anthropology, medicine, odontology, biology, chemistry, documents, engineering, and toxicology. The society sponsors and participates in a wide range of meetings on general and specialized topics in forensic science, such as alcohol and highway safety, bloodstain pattern recognition, and DNA typing and analysis and issues a quarterly publication, *The Journal*, which includes original research papers, reviews, and commentaries on all aspects of forensic science.

Committee on Data for Science and Technology (CODATA)
International Council for Science
URL: http://www.codata.org/
E-mail: codata@dial.oleane.com
Phone: +33 1 45250496
51, Boulevard de Montmorency
75016 Paris
France

The Committee on Data for Science and Technology (CODATA) was established in 1967 as a special committee of the International Council for Science for the purpose of improving the quality, reliability, management, and accessibility of data of importance to all fields of science and technology. One of its many functions has been to analyze and evaluate anthropometric data collected from a variety of sources and for a variety of purposes. It served as one of the primary organizations responsible for the formation of the World Engineering Anthropometric Resources (WEAR) group, some of whose earliest meetings were held in conjunction with CODATA's annual conferences.

Consortium of Forensic Science Organizations (CFSO)
URL: http://www.thecfso.org/
E-mail: press@thecfso.org
Phone: (651) 681-8566
2535 Pilot Knob Road
Mendota Heights, MN 55120-1120

The Consortium of Forensic Science Organizations (CFSO) consists of six specialized forensic science associations, the American Academy of Forensic Sciences, American Society of Crime Laboratory Directors, American Society of Crime Lab Directors—Laboratory Accreditation Board, Forensic Quality Services, International Association for Identification, and National Association of Medical Examiners. The purpose of the organization is to allow members from these organizations to "speak with one voice" on matters that are of concern to those working in the field of forensic science. In order to achieve this goal, CFSO works closely with the National Institute of Justice, the Federal Bureau of Investigation, the Technical Support Working Group, the Department of Homeland Security, the United States Congress, and other governmental agencies.

DNA Academy
URL: http://www.albany.edu/nerfi/dna_academy/
E-mail: nerfi@uamail.albany.edu
Phone: (518) 442-3300

University of Albany
1400 Washington Avenue
Albany, NY 12222

The DNA Academy at the University of Albany's Northeast Regional Forensics Institute was created in 2004 with a grant from the U.S. Department of Justice. The academy offers a customized curriculum in the forensic sciences, state-of-the-art laboratory equipment, a staff of international multilingual instructors with extensive on-the-job experience, and a rapid turnaround time on casework problems.

European Network for Forensic Science Institutes (ENFSI)
URL: http://www.enfsi.eu/
Phone: +31 (0)70 888 61 06
ENFSI Secretariat
P.O. Box 24044
NL2490 AA The Hague
The Netherlands

The European Network for Forensic Science Institutes (ENFSI) was established on October 20, 1995, after three years of preliminary meetings among directors of government forensic laboratories in 11 European governments. The purpose of the organization is to ensure that the quality of technical information in European forensic laboratories is equal to that anywhere in the world. ENFSI currently has working groups in 16 forensic areas, including digital imaging, DNA typing, document investigation, drugs, explosives, fibers, fingerprints, firearms, forensic speech and audio analysis, handwriting analysis, and paint and glass investigation.

Federation of American Scientists (FAS)
URL: http://www.fas.org/main/home.jsp
E-mail: webmaster@fas.org
Phone: (202) 546-3300
1717 K Street, NW
Suite 209
Washington, DC 20036

The Federation of American Scientists (FAS) was formed in 1945 by a group of scientists who had been working on the Manhattan Project to develop the first nuclear weapons. These scientists were very much concerned about the moral consequences of their research and formed FAS to bring to the attention of the general public and the scientific community issues raised by nuclear research. Over the past six decades, the organization has expanded its interests to include a number of other socioscientific issues, such as strategic security, arms trade, biological and chemical weapons, government secrecy, terrorism, weapons in space, information technology for learning and research, and energy and the environment.

Innocence Project
URL: http://www.innocenceproject.org
E-mail: info@innocenceproject.org
Phone: (212) 364-5340
100 Fifth Avenue
3rd Floor
New York, NY 10011

The Innocence Project was established in 1992 at the Benjamin

N. Cardozo School of Law of Yeshiva University in New York City by Barry C. Scheck and Peter J. Neufeld for the purpose of assisting individuals improperly convicted of crimes. The organization bases its advocacy work on DNA evidence that has the likelihood of providing conclusive evidence of a person's innocence. Its cases are conducted by law students who work under the supervision of attorneys and legal staff. As of early 2008, more than 200 individuals had been exonerated of the crimes for which they had been convicted, based on DNA typing evidence.

International Association for Identification (IAI)
URL: http://www.theiai.org
Phone: (651) 681-8566
2535 Pilot Knob Road
Suite 117
Mendota Heights, MN 55120-1120

The International Association for Identification (IAI) claims to be the "oldest and largest forensic organization in the world." It was founded in 1915 at the instigation of Harry H. Caldwell, then an inspector in the Oakland (California) Police Department's Bureau of Identification. The association provides training and certification programs in six fields of forensic identification: bloodstain pattern analysis, crime scene investigation, footwear, forensic art, forensic photography and imaging, and latent print analysis.

International Association of Crime Analysts (IACA)
URL: http://www.iaca.net/
E-mail: iaca@iaca.net
Phone: (800) 609-3419
9218 Metcalf Avenue, #364
Overland Park, Kansas 66212

The International Association of Crime Analysts (IACA) was formed in 1990 for the purpose of helping crime analysts around the world to improve their professional skills and to expedite the exchange of information among members of the profession; to help law enforcement agencies make the best possible use of the skills that crime analysts possess; and to work for improved standards of performance and technique in the profession. The organization currently has about 1,000 members from the United States and about three dozen foreign countries. The organization sponsors an annual conference and offers a variety of courses and workshops dealing with important topics in the field of crime analysis.

International Association of Law Enforcement Intelligence Analysts (IALEIA)
URL: http://www.ialeia.org/
E-mail: admin@ialeia.org
P.O. Box 13857
Richmond, VA 23225

The International Association of Law Enforcement Intelligence Analysts (IALEIA) was formed in 1981 by a group of individuals interested in meeting the special needs of personnel involved in analytical studies in the law enforcement community. The goal of the agency is to "promote standards of excellence in law enforcement analysis by enhancing the mutual exchange of ideas, promoting standards, and providing training." The organization offers special training sessions in the field of analytical studies in law enforcement, an annual conference, and professional awards and scholarships to individuals working in the field.

Scientific Working Group of Friction Ridge Analysis, Study and Technology (SWGFAST)
URL: http://www.swgfast.org/
Orange County Sheriff Coroner
Forensic Science Services
320 North Flower
Santa Ana, CA 92703

The Scientific Working Group of Friction Ridge Analysis, Study and Technology was established in 1997 through the efforts of the Federal Bureau of Investigation and continues to operate under the FBI's sponsorship. SWGFAST's mission is to develop guidelines and procedures for the collection and use of latent fingerprints. The organization has developed and promulgated guidelines for topics such as friction ridge automation training, friction ridge digital imaging, friction ridge examination methodology for latent print examiners, latent print proficiency testing programs, professional conduct, minimum qualifications for latent print trainees, quality assurance guidelines for latent print examiners, and standards for conclusions.

World Engineering Anthropometry Resource (WEAR)
URL: http://ovrt.nist.gov/projects/wear/
Phone: (301) 975-6478
Information Access Division
National Institute of Standards and Technology (NIST)
100 Bureau Drive
Stop 8940
Gaithersburg, MD 208998940

The World Engineering Anthropometry Resource (WEAR) is an international collaborative effort to create a worldwide resource of anthropometric data for a wide variety of engineering applications. WEAR's web site is being hosted by the Visualization and Usability Group of the Information Access Division of the Information Technology Laboratory of the National Institute of Standards and Technology. Other members of the collaborative effort include the U.S. Air Force Research Laboratory, Chonnam University (Korea), the Digital Human Research Center of the National Institute of Advanced Industrial Science and Technology (Japan), UFR Biomedicale des Saints-Pères Laboratoire d'Anthropologie Appliquée of the Université René Descartes (France), National Research Council of Canada, SHARP Dummies Pty Ltd. (Australia), the Delft University of Technology Faculty of Industrial Design Engineering (The Netherlands), Ergonomics Technologies (South Africa), and the Ergonomics Laboratory of the Industrial Design Division of the National Institute of Technology.

PART III

APPENDICES

APPENDIX A

METHODS USED IN BERTILLONAGE (1889)

Alphonse Bertillon developed a very complete system for taking measurements of the human body as a means of identifying possible criminals. He published the instructions for conducting the examinations needed to collect anthropometric data in a number of publications, one of which was *Instructions for Taking Descriptions for the Identification of Criminals and Others by Means of Anthropometric Indications*, published in 1889. That book was translated into English by Gallus Miller and was republished by AMS Press in 1977. In about 80 pages of text and more than 40 diagrams, Bertillon explains in precise detail the measurements to be taken in his system. The diagram below shows his sketches of the basic types of noses an examiner might expect to find.

The Nose

Dimensions
Length (long, medium, short)
Projection (prominent, moderate, slight)
Breadth (broad, medium, narrow)

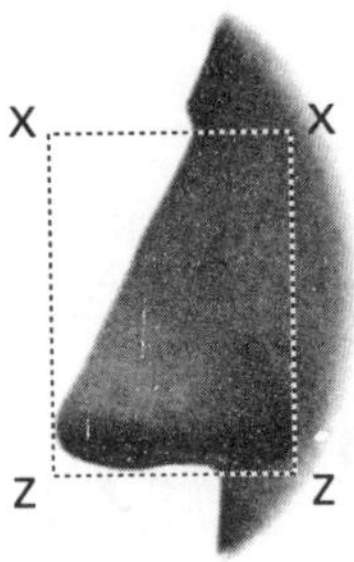

Length X to Z
Projection Z to Z

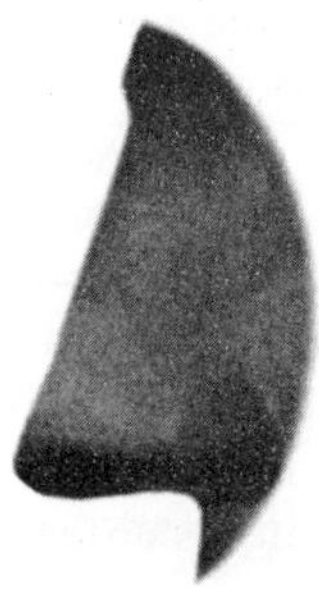

(long, moderately prominent)

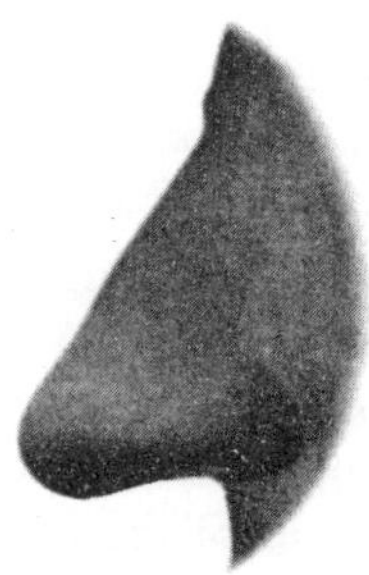

(medium, prominent)

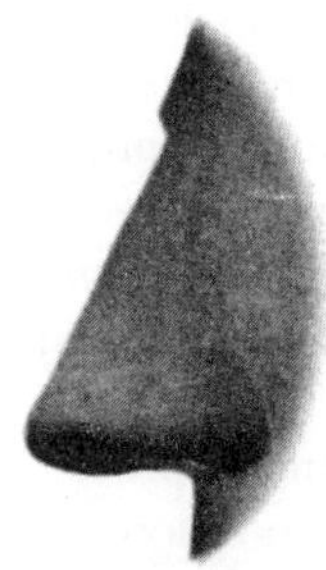

(short, slightly prominent)

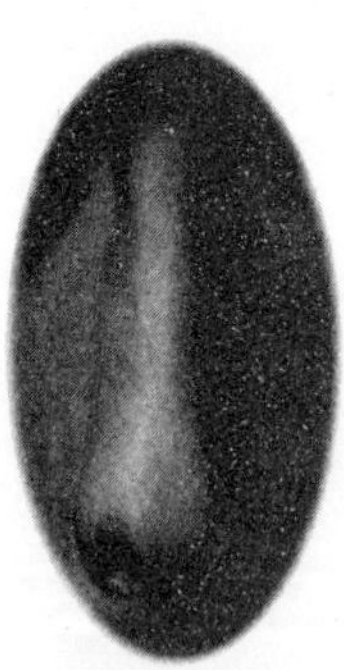

(long, narrow)

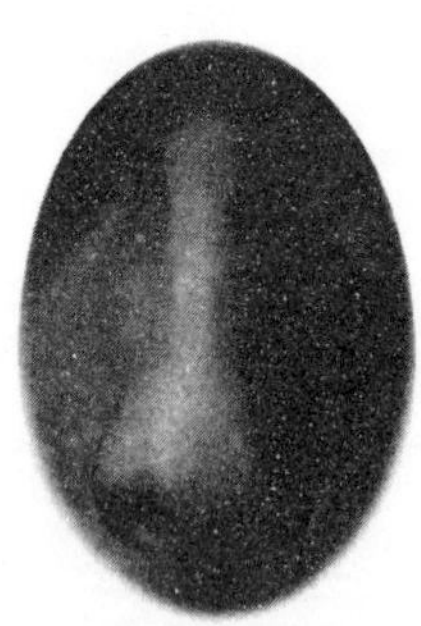

(medium, medium)

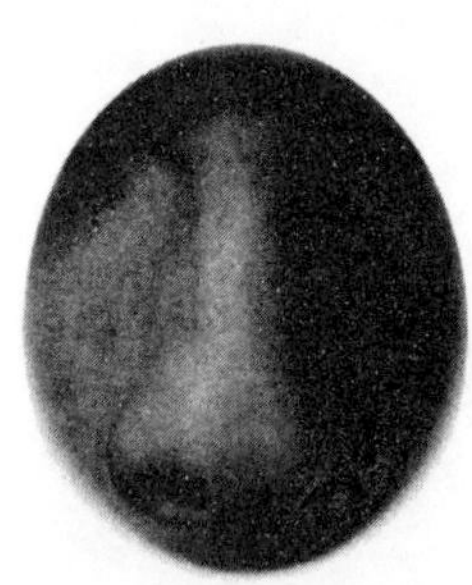

(short, broad)

APPENDIX B

FINGERPRINT PATTERNS

Examiners look for a number of characteristic features in identifying fingerprints. The three most important of those features are loops, whorls, and arches. Each of these features may, in turn, be subdivided into more specific types, such as plain arches and tented arches, plain whorls and double loop whorls, and plain loop and twinned loop. The diagrams below illustrate examples of these six types of fingerprints.

Fingerprint Pattern

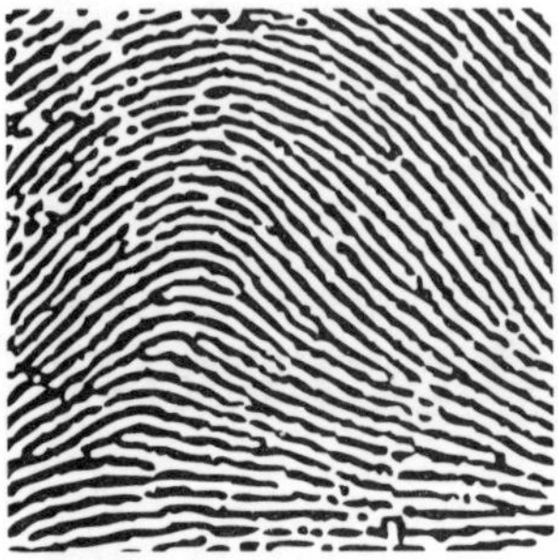

Plain arch

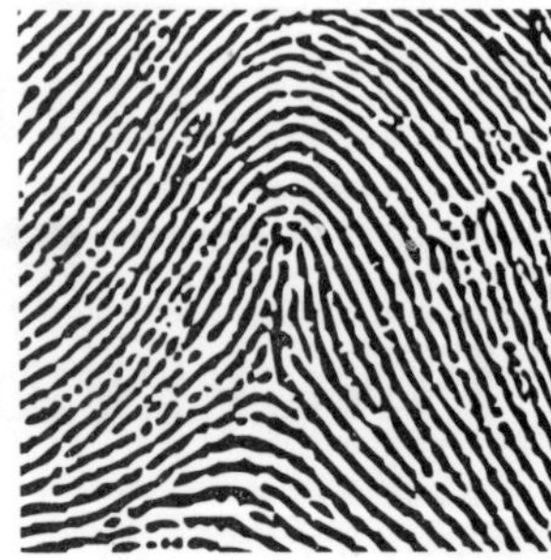

Tented arch

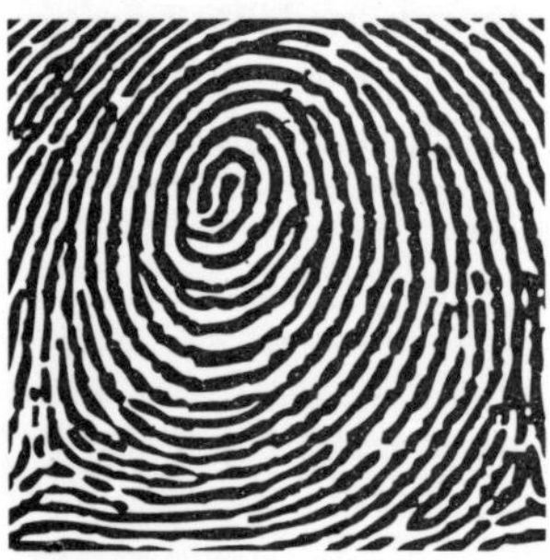

Plain whorl

Double loop whorl

Plain loop

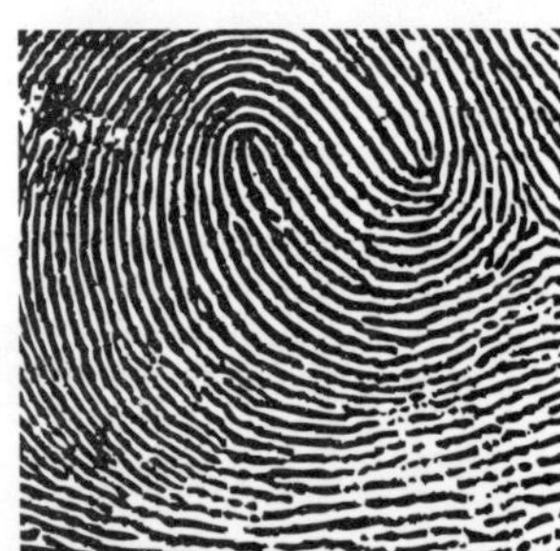

Twinned loop

APPENDIX C

FRYE V. UNITED STATES, ON THE ADMISSIBILITY OF EXPERT TESTIMONY, 1923

Until 1923, federal courts in the United States relied on case law and common law to determine standards for the admissibility of testimony by expert witnesses. Absent a single guiding federal principle, standards varied from district to district and court to court. In 1923, the U.S. Court of Appeals for the District of Columbia received a case in which the primary issue is whether evidence obtained from a particular new forensic technology, polygraph testing, could be admitted to evidence. The court decided that the technology had not yet received general approval within the scientific community, and that, therefore, polygraph evidence could not be considered valid and reliable. The standard for admissibility of expert testimony set by this decision, which became known as the Frye *standard, remained the primary criterion for the admissibility of expert testimony for 70 years in the United States.*

Frye v. United States
54 App. D. C. 46, 293 F. 1013
No. 3968
Court of Appeals of District of Columbia
Submitted November 7, 1923
Decided December 3, 1923

Before SMYTH, Chief Justice, VAN ORSDEL, Associate Justice, and MARTIN, Presiding Judge of the United States Court of Customs Appeals.

VAN ORSDEL, Associate Justice. Appellant, defendant below, was convicted of the crime of murder in the second degree, and from the judgment prosecutes this appeal.

A single assignment of error is presented for our consideration. In the course of the trial counsel for defendant offered an expert witness to testify to the result of a deception test made upon defendant. The test is described as the systolic blood pressure deception test. It is asserted that blood pressure is influenced by change in the emotions of the witness, and that the systolic blood pressure rises are brought about by nervous impulses sent to the sympathetic branch of the autonomic nervous system. Scientific experiments, it is claimed, have demonstrated that fear, rage, and pain always produce a rise of systolic blood pressure, and that conscious deception or falsehood, concealment of facts, or guilt of crime, accompanied by fear of detection when the person is under examination, raises the systolic blood pressure in a curve, which corresponds exactly to the struggle going on in the subject's mind, between fear and attempted control of that fear, as the examination touches the vital points in respect of which he is attempting to deceive the examiner.

In other words, the theory seems to be that truth is spontaneous, and comes without conscious effort, while the utterance of a falsehood requires a conscious effort, which is reflected in the blood pressure. The rise thus produced is easily detected and distinguished from the rise produced by mere fear of the examination itself. In the former instance, the pressure rises higher than in the latter, and is more pronounced as the examination proceeds, while in the latter case, if the subject is telling the truth, the pressure registers highest at the beginning of the examination, and gradually diminishes as the examination proceeds.

Prior to the trial defendant was subjected to this deception test, and counsel offered the scientist who conducted the test as an expert to testify to the results obtained. The offer was objected to by counsel for the government, and the court sustained the objection. Counsel for defendant then offered to have the proffered witness conduct a test in the presence of the jury. This also was denied.

Counsel for defendant, in their able presentation of the novel question involved, correctly state in their brief that no cases directly in point have been found. The broad ground, however, upon which they plant their case, is succinctly stated in their brief as follows:

> *"The rule is that the opinions of experts or skilled witnesses are admissible in evidence in those cases in which the matter of inquiry is such that inexperienced persons are unlikely to prove capable of forming a correct judgment upon it, for the reason that the subject-matter so far partakes of a science, art, or trade as to require a previous habit or experience or study in it, in order to acquire a knowledge of it. When the question involved does not lie within the range of common experience or common knowledge, but requires special experience or special knowledge, then the opinions of witnesses skilled in that particular science, art, or trade to which the question relates are admissible in evidence."*

Numerous cases are cited in support of this rule. Just when a scientific principle or discovery crosses the line between the experimental and demonstrable stages is difficult to define. Somewhere in this twilight zone the evidential force of the principle must be recognized, and while courts will go a long way in admitting expert testimony deduced from a well-recognized scientific principle or discovery, the thing from which the deduction is made must be sufficiently established to have gained general acceptance in the particular field in which it belongs.

We think the systolic blood pressure deception test has not yet gained such standing and scientific recognition among physiological and psychological authorities as would justify the courts in admitting expert testimony deduced from the discovery, development, and experiments thus far made.

The judgment is affirmed.

APPENDIX D

EMPLOYEE POLYGRAPH PROTECTION ACT OF 1988

In 1988 Congress passed the Employee Polygraph Protection Act, setting out limitations on the use of various lie detector devices for purposes of hiring and/or retaining employees. The act is now codified in the United States Code, Title 29, Chapter 22. Some relevant sections of the code are reprinted below.

§ 2001. Definitions

. . .

(2) Employer

The term "employer" includes any person acting directly or indirectly in the interest of an employer in relation to an employee or prospective employee.

(3) Lie detector

The term "lie detector" includes a polygraph, deceptograph, voice stress analyzer, psychological stress evaluator, or any other similar device (whether mechanical or electrical) that is used, or the results of which are used, for the purpose of rendering a diagnostic opinion regarding the honesty or dishonesty of an individual.

(4) Polygraph

The term "polygraph" means an instrument that—

(A) records continuously, visually, permanently, and simultaneously changes in cardiovascular, respiratory, and electrodermal patterns as minimum instrumentation standards; and

(B) is used, or the results of which are used, for the purpose of rendering a diagnostic opinion regarding the honesty or dishonesty of an individual.

§ 2002. Prohibitions on lie detector use

Except as provided in sections 2006 and 2007 of this title, it shall be unlawful for any employer engaged in or affecting commerce or in the production of goods for commerce—

(1) directly or indirectly, to require, request, suggest, or cause any employee or prospective employee to take or submit to any lie detector test;
(2) to use, accept, refer to, or inquire concerning the results of any lie detector test of any employee or prospective employee;
(3) to discharge, discipline, discriminate against in any manner, or deny employment or promotion to, or threaten to take any such action against—
(A) any employee or prospective employee who refuses, declines, or fails to take or submit to any lie detector test, or
(B) any employee or prospective employee on the basis of the results of any lie detector test; or
(4) to discharge, discipline, discriminate against in any manner, or deny employment or promotion to, or threaten to take any such action against, any employee or prospective employee because—
(A) such employee or prospective employee has filed any complaint or instituted or caused to be instituted any proceeding under or related to this chapter,
(B) such employee or prospective employee has testified or is about to testify in any such proceeding, or
(C) of the exercise by such employee or prospective employee, on behalf of such employee or another person, of any right afforded by this chapter.
. . .

§ 2006. Exemptions
(a) No application to governmental employers
This chapter shall not apply with respect to the United States Government, any State or local government, or any political subdivision of a State or local government.
(b) National defense and security exemption
(1) National defense
Nothing in this chapter shall be construed to prohibit the administration, by the Federal Government, in the performance of any counterintelligence function, of any lie detector test to—
(A) any expert or consultant under contract to the Department of Defense or any employee of any contractor of such Department; or
(B) any expert or consultant under contract with the Department of Energy in connection with the atomic energy defense activities of such Department or any employee of any contractor of such Department in connection with such activities.
(2) Security
Nothing in this chapter shall be construed to prohibit the administration, by the Federal Government, in the performance of any intelligence or counterintelligence function, of any lie detector test to—

(A)
(i) any individual employed by, assigned to, or detailed to, the National Security Agency, the Defense Intelligence Agency, the National Geospatial-Intelligence Agency, or the Central Intelligence Agency,
(ii) any expert or consultant under contract to any such agency,
(iii) any employee of a contractor to any such agency,
(iv) any individual applying for a position in any such agency, or
(v) any individual assigned to a space where sensitive cryptologic information is produced, processed, or stored for any such agency; or
(B) any expert, or consultant (or employee of such expert or consultant) under contract with any Federal Government department, agency, or program whose duties involve access to information that has been classified at the level of top secret or designated as being within a special access program under section 4.2(a) of Executive Order 12356 (or a successor Executive order).
(c) FBI contractors exemption
Nothing in this chapter shall be construed to prohibit the administration, by the Federal Government, in the performance of any counterintelligence function, of any lie detector test to an employee of a contractor of the Federal Bureau of Investigation of the Department of Justice who is engaged in the performance of any work under the contract with such Bureau.
(d) Limited exemption for ongoing investigations
[This section lists a number of special cases and circumstances under which polygraph testing is permitted provided that certain specific conditions are met. Two examples are included.]
. . .

(1) the test is administered in connection with an ongoing investigation involving economic loss or injury to the employer's business, such as theft, embezzlement, misappropriation, or an act of unlawful industrial espionage or sabotage; *[and other conditions are met]*
. . .

. . . this chapter shall not prohibit the use of polygraph tests on prospective employees by any private employer whose primary business purpose consists of providing armored car personnel, personnel engaged in the design, installation, and maintenance of security alarm systems, or other uniformed or plainclothes security personnel and whose function includes protection of—
(A) facilities, materials, or operations having a significant impact on the health or safety of any State or political subdivision thereof, or the national security of the United States, as determined under rules and regulations issued by the Secretary within 90 days after June 27, 1988, including— *[special provisions follow.]*

APPENDIX E

POLYGRAPH TESTING, U.S. MILITARY RULES OF EVIDENCE, RULE 707 (1991)

In 1991, President George H. W. Bush authorized an addition to the Military Rules of Evidence dealing with the use of evidence collected from polygraph testing. That rule, known as Rule 707, was tested and declared constitutional by the U.S. Supreme Court in the case of United States v. Scheffer *in 1996. The rule is given in its entirety below.*

Rule 707. Polygraph Examinations
(a) Notwithstanding any other provision of law, the results of a polygraph examination, the opinion of a polygraph examiner, or any reference to an offer to take, failure to take, or taking of a polygraph examination, shall not be admitted into evidence.
(b) Nothing in this section is intended to exclude from evidence statements made during a polygraph examination which are otherwise admissible.

APPENDIX F

DAUBERT V. MERRELL, ON THE ADMISSIBILITY OF EXPERT TESTIMONY, 1993

In 1993, the U.S. Supreme Court heard testimony on a case in which questions were raised as to the admissibility of scientific evidence presented by the defense. At stake was the question as to whether a previous standard, Frye v. United States, *decided in 1923, or the Federal Rules of Evidence (FRE), adopted in 1975, held priority in deciding the status of evidence. The Court held that FRE was to be taken as the standard for admissibility of evidence, in preference to the* Frye *standard. The case has been called by legal experts one of the most important legal decisions in the United States in the 20th century.*

DAUBERT et ux., individually and as guardians and litem for DAUBERT, et al. v. MERRELL DOW PHARMACEUTICALS, INC.

certiorari to the united states court of appeals for the ninth circuit

No. 92102. Argued March 30, 1993—Decided June 28, 1993

Petitioners, two minor children and their parents, alleged in their suit against respondent that the children's serious birth defects had been caused by the mothers' prenatal ingestion of Bendectin, a prescription drug marketed by respondent. The District Court granted respondent summary judgment based on a well credentialed expert's affidavit concluding, upon reviewing the extensive published scientific literature on the subject, that maternal use of Bendectin has not been shown to be a risk factor for human birth defects. Although petitioners had responded with the testimony of eight other well credentialed experts, who based their conclusion that Bendectin can cause birth defects on animal studies, chemical structure analyses, and the unpublished "reanalysis" of previously published human statistical studies, the court determined that this evidence did not meet the applicable "general acceptance" standard for the admission of expert testimony. The Court of Appeals agreed and affirmed, citing *Frye v. United States*, 54 App. D. C. 46, 47, 293 F. 1013, 1014, for the rule that expert opinion based on a scientific technique is inadmissible unless the technique is "generally accepted" as reliable in the relevant scientific community.

Held: The Federal Rules of Evidence, not Frye, provide the standard for admitting expert scientific testimony in a federal trial. Pp. 417.

(a) Frye's "general acceptance" test was superseded by the Rules' adoption. The Rules occupy the field, United States v. Abel, 469 U.S. 45, 49, and, although the common law of evidence may serve as an aid to their application, id., at 5152, respondent's assertion that they somehow assimilated Frye is unconvincing. Nothing in the Rules as a whole or in the text and drafting history of Rule 702, which specifically governs expert testimony, gives any indication that "general acceptance" is a necessary precondition to the admissibility of scientific evidence. Moreover, such a rigid standard would be at odds with the Rules' liberal thrust and their general approach of relaxing the traditional barriers to "opinion" testimony. Pp. 4–8.

(b) The Rules—especially Rule 702—place appropriate limits on the admissibility of purportedly scientific evidence by assigning to the trial judge the task of ensuring that an expert's testimony both rests on a reliable foundation and is relevant to the task at hand. The reliability standard is established by Rule 702's requirement that an expert's testimony pertain to "scientific . . . knowledge," since the adjective "scientific" implies a grounding in science's methods and procedures, while the word "knowledge" connotes a body of known facts or of ideas inferred from such facts or accepted as true on good grounds. The Rule's requirement that the testimony "assist the trier of fact to understand the evidence or to determine a fact in issue" goes primarily to relevance by demanding a valid scientific connection to the pertinent inquiry as a precondition to admissibility. Pp. 9–12.

(c) Faced with a proffer of expert scientific testimony under Rule 702, the trial judge, pursuant to Rule 104(a), must make a preliminary assessment of whether the testimony's underlying reasoning or methodology is scientifically valid and properly can be applied to the facts at issue. Many considerations will bear on the inquiry, including whether the theory or technique in question can be (and has been) tested, whether it has been subjected to peer review and publication, its known or potential error rate, and the existence and maintenance of standards controlling its operation, and whether it has attracted widespread acceptance within a relevant scientific community. The inquiry is a flexible one, and its focus must be solely on principles and methodology, not on the conclusions that they generate. Throughout, the judge should also be mindful of other applicable Rules. Pp. 12–15.

(d) Cross-examination, presentation of contrary evidence, and careful instruction on the burden of proof, rather than wholesale exclusion under an uncompromising "general acceptance" standard, is the appropriate means by which evidence based on valid principles may be challenged. That even limited screening by the trial judge, on occasion, will prevent the jury from hearing of authentic scientific breakthroughs is simply a consequence of the fact that the Rules are not designed to seek cosmic understanding but, rather, to resolve legal disputes. Pp. 15–17.

951 F. 2d 1128, vacated and remanded.

Blackmun, J., delivered the opinion for a unanimous Court with respect to Parts I and IIA, and the opinion of the Court with respect to Parts IIB, IIC, III, and IV, in which White, O'Connor, Scalia, Kennedy, Souter, and Thomas, JJ., joined. Rehnquist, C. J., filed an opinion concurring in part and dissenting in part, in which Stevens, J., joined.

APPENDIX G

STATUTORY REQUIREMENTS FOR DNA TESTING (1994)

In 1994, Congress passed amendments to the Omnibus Crime Control and Safe Streets Act of 1968 that contained three sections dealing with DNA testing. Those three sections provided for the monitoring of forensic laboratories in which DNA typing was carried out, provided for the creation of a national index containing DNA samples, and described specific requirements for members of the Federal Bureau of Investigation (FBI) who were involved in DNA testing. Important sections of that act are excerpted below.

§ 14131. QUALITY ASSURANCE AND PROFICIENCY TESTING STANDARDS

(a) Publication of quality assurance and proficiency testing standards
(1)
(A) Not later than 180 days after September 13, 1994, the Director of the Federal Bureau of Investigation shall appoint an advisory board on DNA quality assurance methods from among nominations proposed by the head of the National Academy of Sciences and professional societies of crime laboratory officials.
(B) The advisory board shall include as members scientists from State, local, and private forensic laboratories, molecular geneticists and population geneticists not affiliated with a forensic laboratory, and a representative from the National Institute of Standards and Technology.
(C) The advisory board shall develop, and if appropriate, periodically revise, recommended standards for quality assurance, including standards for testing the proficiency of forensic laboratories, and forensic analysts, in conducting analyses of DNA.
(2) The Director of the Federal Bureau of Investigation, after taking into consideration such recommended standards, shall issue (and revise from time to time) standards for quality assurance, including standards for testing

the proficiency of forensic laboratories, and forensic analysts, in conducting analyses of DNA.

(3) The standards described in paragraphs (1) and (2) shall specify criteria for quality assurance and proficiency tests to be applied to the various types of DNA analyses used by forensic laboratories. The standards shall also include a system for grading proficiency testing performance to determine whether a laboratory is performing acceptably.

(4) Until such time as the advisory board has made recommendations to the Director of the Federal Bureau of Investigation and the Director has acted upon those recommendations, the quality assurance guidelines adopted by the technical working group on DNA analysis methods shall be deemed the Director's standards for purposes of this section.

. . .

(c) Proficiency testing program

(1) Not later than 1 year after the effective date of this Act, the Director of the National Institute of Justice shall certify to the Committees on the Judiciary of the House and Senate that—

(A) the Institute has entered into a contract with, or made a grant to, an appropriate entity for establishing, or has taken other appropriate action to ensure that there is established, not later than 2 years after September 13, 1994, a blind external proficiency testing program for DNA analyses, which shall be available to public and private laboratories performing forensic DNA analyses;

(B) a blind external proficiency testing program for DNA analyses is already readily available to public and private laboratories performing forensic DNA analyses; or

(C) it is not feasible to have blind external testing for DNA forensic analyses.

(2) As used in this subsection, the term "blind external proficiency test" means a test that is presented to a forensic laboratory through a second agency and appears to the analysts to involve routine evidence.

. . .

§ 14132. Index to Facilitate Law Enforcement Exchange of DNA Identification Information

(a) Establishment of index

The Director of the Federal Bureau of Investigation may establish an index of—

(1) DNA identification records of persons convicted of crimes;

(2) analyses of DNA samples recovered from crime scenes;

(3) analyses of DNA samples recovered from unidentified human remains; and

(4) analyses of DNA samples voluntarily contributed from relatives of missing persons.

(b) Information

The index described in subsection (a) of this section shall include only information on DNA identification records and DNA analyses that are—

(1) based on analyses performed by or on behalf of a criminal justice agency (or the Secretary of Defense in accordance with section 1565 of title 10) in accordance with publicly available standards that satisfy or exceed the guidelines for a quality assurance program for DNA analysis, issued by the Director of the Federal Bureau of Investigation under section 14131 of this title;

(2) prepared by laboratories, and DNA analysts, that undergo semiannual external proficiency testing by a DNA proficiency testing program meeting the standards issued under section 14131 of this title; and

(3) maintained by Federal, State, and local criminal justice agencies (or the Secretary of Defense in accordance with section 1565 of title 10) pursuant to rules that allow disclosure of stored DNA samples and DNA analyses only—

(A) to criminal justice agencies for law enforcement identification purposes;

(B) in judicial proceedings, if otherwise admissible pursuant to applicable statutes or rules;

(C) for criminal defense purposes, to a defendant, who shall have access to samples and analyses performed in connection with the case in which such defendant is charged; or

(D) if personally identifiable information is removed, for a population statistics database, for identification research and protocol development purposes, or for quality control purposes.

(c) Failure to comply

Access to the index established by this section is subject to cancellation if the quality control and privacy requirements described in subsection (b) of this section are not met.

(d) Expungement of records

(1) By Director

(A) The Director of the Federal Bureau of Investigation shall promptly expunge from the index described in subsection (a) of this section the DNA analysis of a person included in the index on the basis of a qualifying Federal offense or a qualifying District of Columbia offense (as determined under sections 14135a and 14135b of this title, respectively) if the Director receives, for each conviction of the person of a qualifying offense, a certified copy of a final court order establishing that such conviction has been overturned.

. . .

(2) By States
(A) As a condition of access to the index described in subsection (a) of this section, a State shall promptly expunge from that index the DNA analysis of a person included in the index by that State if the responsible agency or official of that State receives, for each conviction of the person of an offense on the basis of which that analysis was or could have been included in the index, a certified copy of a final court order establishing that such conviction has been overturned.
. . .

§ 14133. FEDERAL BUREAU OF INVESTIGATION

(a) Proficiency testing requirements
(1) Generally
(A) Personnel at the Federal Bureau of Investigation who perform DNA analyses shall undergo semiannual external proficiency testing by a DNA proficiency testing program meeting the standards issued under section 14131 of this title.
(B) Within 1 year after September 13, 1994, the Director of the Federal Bureau of Investigation shall arrange for periodic blind external tests to determine the proficiency of DNA analysis performed at the Federal Bureau of Investigation laboratory.
(C) In this paragraph, "blind external test" means a test that is presented to the laboratory through a second agency and appears to the analysts to involve routine evidence.
. . .
(b) Privacy protection standards
(1) Generally
Except as provided in paragraph (2), the results of DNA tests performed for a Federal law enforcement agency for law enforcement purposes may be disclosed only—
(A) to criminal justice agencies for law enforcement identification purposes;
(B) in judicial proceedings, if otherwise admissible pursuant to applicable statues [1] or rules; and
(C) for criminal defense purposes, to a defendant, who shall have access to samples and analyses performed in connection with the case in which such defendant is charged.
(2) Exception
[This section lists certain exceptions to the preceding section.]
(2) A person who, without authorization, knowingly obtains DNA samples or individually identifiable DNA information indexed in a database created or maintained by any Federal law enforcement agency shall be fined not more than $100,000.

APPENDIX H

UNITED STATES V. SCHEFFER ON THE ADMISSIBILITY OF POLYGRAPH TEST RESULTS, 1998

United States v. Scheffer *dealt with the question as to whether a defendant has the right to submit evidence obtained during polygraph testing in his or her own defense. That question is very closely tied to the question of scientific acceptance of polygraph testing. The Court pointed out that the ability to offer evidence in one's own defense depends at least partially on the relevance and validity of that evidence. In this case, the U.S. Supreme Court ruled that polygraph testing had not yet attained a level of broad acceptance in the scientific community and that, therefore, the defendant was not entitled to use the evidence in his own defense.*

A defendant's right to present relevant evidence is not unlimited, but rather is subject to reasonable restrictions.* A defendant's interest in presenting such evidence may thus " 'bow to accommodate other legitimate interests in the criminal trial process.' " As a result, state and federal rulemakers have broad latitude under the Constitution to establish rules excluding evidence from criminal trials. Such rules do not abridge an accused's right to present a defense so long as they are not "arbitrary" or "disproportionate to the purposes they are designed to serve." Moreover, we have found the exclusion of evidence to be unconstitutionally arbitrary or disproportionate only where it has infringed upon a weighty interest of the accused.

Rule 707** serves several legitimate interests in the criminal trial process. These interests include ensuring that only reliable evidence is introduced at trial, preserving the jury's role in determining credibility, and avoiding litigation that is collateral to the primary purpose of the trial. The rule is neither arbitrary nor disproportionate in promoting these ends. Nor does it implicate a sufficiently weighty interest of the defendant to raise a constitutional concern under our precedents.

A

State and federal governments unquestionably have a legitimate interest in ensuring that reliable evidence is presented to the trier of fact in a criminal trial. Indeed, the exclusion of unreliable evidence is a principal objective of many evidentiary rules.

The contentions of respondent and the dissent notwithstanding, there is simply no consensus that polygraph evidence is reliable. To this day, the scientific community remains extremely polarized about the reliability of polygraph techniques. Some studies have concluded that polygraph tests overall are accurate and reliable. Others have found that polygraph tests assess truthfulness significantly less accurately—that scientific field studies suggest the accuracy rate of the "control question technique" polygraph is "little better than could be obtained by the toss of a coin," that is, 50 percent.

This lack of scientific consensus is reflected in the disagreement among state and federal courts concerning both the admissibility and the reliability of polygraph evidence. Although some Federal Courts of Appeal have abandoned the per se rule excluding polygraph evidence, leaving its admission or exclusion to the discretion of district courts under Daubert,*** at least one Federal Circuit has recently reaffirmed its per se ban . . . and another recently noted that it has "not decided whether polygraphy has reached a sufficient state of reliability to be admissible." Most States maintain per se rules excluding polygraph evidence. New Mexico is unique in making polygraph evidence generally admissible without the prior stipulation of the parties and without significant restriction. Whatever their approach, state and federal courts continue to express doubt about whether such evidence is reliable.

The approach taken by the President in adopting Rule 707—excluding polygraph evidence in all military trials—is a rational and proportional means of advancing the legitimate interest in barring unreliable evidence. Although the degree of reliability of polygraph evidence may depend upon a variety of identifiable factors, there is simply no way to know in a particular case whether a polygraph examiner's conclusion is accurate, because certain doubts and uncertainties plague even the best polygraph exams. Individual jurisdictions therefore may reasonably reach differing conclusions as to whether polygraph evidence should be admitted. We cannot say, then, that presented with such widespread uncertainty, the President acted arbitrarily or disproportionately in promulgating a per se rule excluding all polygraph evidence.

B

It is equally clear that Rule 707 serves a second legitimate governmental interest: Preserving the jury's core function of making credibility determinations in criminal trials. A fundamental premise of our criminal trial system is that "the jury is the lie detector." Determining the weight and credibility of witness testimony, therefore, has long been held to be the "part of every case [that] belongs to the jury, who are presumed to be fitted for it by their natural intelligence and their practical knowledge of men and the ways of men."

By its very nature, polygraph evidence may diminish the jury's role in making credibility determinations. The common form of polygraph test measures a variety of physiological responses to a set of questions asked by the examiner, who then interprets these physiological correlates of anxiety and offers an opinion to the jury about whether the witness—often, as in this case, the accused—was deceptive in answering questions about the very matters at issue in the trial. Unlike other expert witnesses who testify about factual matters outside the jurors' knowledge, such as the analysis of fingerprints, ballistics, or DNA found at a crime scene, a polygraph expert can supply the jury only with another opinion, in addition to its own, about whether the witness was telling the truth. Jurisdictions, in promulgating rules of evidence, may legitimately be concerned about the risk that juries will give excessive weight to the opinions of a polygrapher, clothed as they are in scientific expertise and at times offering, as in respondent's case, a conclusion about the ultimate issue in the trial. Such jurisdictions may legitimately determine that the aura of infallibility attending polygraph evidence can lead jurors to abandon their duty to assess credibility and guilt. Those jurisdictions may also take into account the fact that a judge cannot determine, when ruling on a motion to admit polygraph evidence, whether a particular polygraph expert is likely to influence the jury unduly. For these reasons, the President is within his constitutional prerogative to promulgate a per se rule that simply excludes all such evidence.

C

A third legitimate interest served by Rule 707 is avoiding litigation over issues other than the guilt or innocence of the accused. Such collateral litigation prolongs criminal trials and threatens to distract the jury from its central function of determining guilt or innocence. Allowing proffers of polygraph evidence would inevitably entail assessments of such issues as whether the test and control questions were appropriate, whether a particular polygraph examiner was qualified and had properly interpreted the physiological responses, and whether other factors such as countermeasures employed by the examinee had distorted the exam results. Such assessments would be required in each and every case. It thus offends no constitutional principle for the President to conclude that a per se rule excluding all polygraph evidence is appropriate. Because litigation over the admissibility of polygraph evidence is by its very nature collateral, a per se rule prohibiting its admission is not an arbitrary or disproportionate means of avoiding it.

---

*Citations omitted from this selection.

**Military Rule of Evidence 707 makes polygraph evidence inadmissible in court-martial proceedings.

***Daubert v. Merrell Dow Pharmaceuticals* (1993), 509 U.S. 579

APPENDIX I

State Laws Concerned with Ballistic Fingerprinting (2000)

In 2000, two states, Maryland and New York, passed legislation requiring new handguns sold in the state to be "fingerprinted." Those ballistic fingerprints were then to be sent to state law enforcement agencies, where they were to become part of a state database for use in solving violent crimes. The complete texts of those two laws are provided below.

MARYLAND LAW

Public Safety
§ 5131.

(a) (1) In this section the following words have the meanings indicated.

(2) "Manufacturer" means a person who possesses a federal license to engage in the business of manufacturing firearms or ammunition for sale or distribution.

(3) "Projectile" means the part of handgun ammunition that is expelled through the barrel of the handgun by an explosion.

(4) "Shell casing" means the part of handgun ammunition that contains the primer and propellent powder to discharge the projectile.

(b) A manufacturer that ships or transports a handgun for sale, rental, or transfer in the State shall include in the box with the handgun in a separate, sealed container:

(1) a shell casing of a projectile discharged from the handgun; and

(2) additional information that the Secretary requires to identify the type of handgun and shell casing.

(c) (1) On receipt of a handgun from a manufacturer, the dealer shall confirm to the Department of State Police that the manufacturer has complied with subsection (b) of this section.

(2) On the sale, rental, or transfer of the handgun, the dealer shall forward the sealed container to the Department of State Police Crime Laboratory.

(d) On receipt of a shell casing and information as required in subsection (b) of this section, the Department of State Police Crime Laboratory shall enter the information in each relevant database.

NEW YORK LAW

Section 396ff. Pistol and revolver ballistic identification databank.

(1) For the purposes of this section, the following terms shall have the following meanings:

(a) "Manufacturer" means any person, firm or corporation possessing a valid federal license that permits such person, firm or corporation to engage in the business of manufacturing pistols or revolvers or ammunition therefor for the purpose of sale or distribution.

(b) "Shell casing" means that part of ammunition capable of being used in a pistol or revolver that contains the primer and propellant powder to discharge the bullet or projectile.

(2) On and after March first, two thousand one, any manufacturer that ships, transports or delivers a pistol or revolver to any person in this state shall, in accordance with rules and regulations promulgated by the division of state police, include in the container with such pistol or revolver a separate sealed container that encloses:

(a) a shell casing of a bullet or projectile discharged from such pistol or revolver; and

(b) any additional information that identifies such pistol or revolver and shell casing as required by such rules and regulations.

(3) A gunsmith or dealer in firearms licensed in this state shall, within ten days of the receipt of any pistol or revolver from a manufacturer that fails to comply with the provisions of this section, either (a) return such pistol or revolver to such manufacturer, or (b) notify the division of state police of such noncompliance and thereafter obtain a substitute sealed container through participation in a program operated by the state police as provided in subdivision four of this section.

(4) The division of state police shall no later than October first, two thousand, promulgate rules and regulations for the operation of a program which provides a gunsmith or a dealer in firearms licensed in this state with

a sealed container enclosing the items specified in subdivision two of this section. The program shall at a minimum:

(a) be operational by January first, two thousand one;

(b) operate in at least five regional locations within the state; and

(c) specify procedures by which such gunsmith or dealer is to deliver a pistol or revolver to the regional program location closest to his or her place of business for testing and prompt return of such pistol or revolver.

(5) On and after March first, two thousand one, a gunsmith or dealer in firearms licensed in this state shall, within ten days of delivering to any person a pistol or revolver received by such gunsmith or dealer in firearms on or after such date, forward to the division of state police, along with the original transaction report required by subdivision twelve of section 400.00 of the penal law, the sealed container enclosing the shell casing from such pistol or revolver either (a) received from the manufacturer, or (b) obtained through participation in the program operated by the division of state police in accordance with subdivision four of this section.

(6) Upon receipt of the sealed container, the division of state police shall cause to be entered in an automated electronic databank pertinent data and other ballistic information relevant to identification of the shell casing and to the pistol or revolver from which it was discharged. The automated electronic databank will be operated and maintained by the division of state police, in accordance with its rules and regulations adopted after consultation with the Federal Bureau of Investigation and the United States Department of Treasury, Bureau of Alcohol, Tobacco and Firearms to ensure compatibility with national ballistic technology.

(7) Any person, firm or corporation who knowingly violates any of the provisions of this section shall be guilty of a violation, punishable as provided in the penal law. Any person, firm or corporation who knowingly violates any of the provisions of this section after having been previously convicted of a violation of this section shall be guilty of a class A misdemeanor, punishable as provided in the penal law.

APPENDIX J

BALLISTICS, LAW ASSISTANCE, AND SAFETY TECHNOLOGY ACT (2002)

Some forensic scientists and law enforcement officials believe that a database containing ballistic records for all weapons used in the United States could be a significant aid in solving many violent crimes. From time to time, legislation to create such a database has been introduced into the U.S. Congress. Perhaps the best known legislation was Senate bill S. 3096 and H.R. 5663, both introduced into the 107th Congress in 2002. The two bills are identical in wording, and the text of the House version is provided here.

107TH CONGRESS
2D SESSION

H. R. 5663

IN THE HOUSE OF REPRESENTATIVES
OCTOBER 16, 2002
Ms. ESHOO (for herself and Mr. CONYERS) introduced the following bill; which
was referred to the Committee on the Judiciary
A BILL

To amend chapter 44 of title 18, United States Code, to require ballistics testing of all firearms manufactured and all firearms in custody of Federal agencies.

Be it enacted by the Senate and House of Representatives of the United States of America in Congress assembled,

Appendix J

SECTION 1. SHORT TITLE.

This Act may be cited as the "Ballistics, Law Assistance, and Safety Technology Act" or the "BLAST Act."

SEC. 2. PURPOSES.

The purposes of this Act are—

(1) to increase public safety by assisting law enforcement in solving more gun-related crimes and offering prosecutors evidence to link felons to gun crimes through ballistics technology;

(2) to provide for ballistics testing of all new firearms for sale to assist in the identification of firearms used in crimes;

(3) to require ballistics testing of all firearms in custody of Federal agencies to assist in the identification of firearms used in crimes; and

(4) to add ballistics testing to existing firearms enforcement programs.

SEC. 3. DEFINITION OF BALLISTICS.

Section 921(a) of title 18, United States Code, is amended by adding at the end the following:

"(35) BALLISTICS.—The term 'ballistics' means a comparative analysis of fired bullets and cartridge casings to identify the firearm from which bullets and cartridge casings were discharged, through identification of the unique characteristics that each firearm imprints on bullets and cartridge casings."

SEC. 4. TEST FIRING AND AUTOMATED STORAGE OF BALLISTICS RECORDS.

(a) AMENDMENT.—Section 923 of title 18, United States Code, is amended by adding at the end the following:

"(m)(1) In addition to the other licensing requirements under this section, a licensed manufacturer or licensed importer shall—

"(A) test fire firearms manufactured or imported by such licensees as specified by the Secretary by regulation;

"(B) prepare ballistics images of the fired bullet and cartridge casings from the test fire;

"(C) make the records available to the Secretary for entry in a computerized database; and

"(D) store the fired bullet and cartridge casings in such a manner and for such a period as specified by the Secretary by regulation.

"(2) Nothing in this subsection creates a cause of action against any Federal firearms licensee or any other person for any civil liability except for imposition of a civil penalty under this section.

"(3)(A) The Attorney General and the Secretary shall assist firearm manufacturers and importers in complying with paragraph (1) through—

"(i) the acquisition, disposition, and upgrades of ballistics equipment and bullet and cartridge casing recovery equipment to be placed at or near the sites of licensed manufacturers and importers;

"(ii) the hiring or designation of personnel necessary to develop and maintain a database of ballistics images of fired bullets and cartridge casings, research and evaluation;

"(iii) providing education about the role of ballistics as part of a comprehensive firearm crime reduction strategy;

"(iv) providing for the coordination among Federal, State, and local law enforcement and regulatory agencies and the firearm industry to curb firearm-related crime and illegal firearm trafficking; and

"(v) any other steps necessary to make ballistics testing effective.

"(B) The Attorney General and the Secretary shall—

"(i) establish a computer system through which State and local law enforcement agencies can promptly access ballistics records stored under this subsection, as soon as such a capability is available; and

"(ii) encourage training for all ballistics examiners.

"(4) Not later than 1 year after the date of enactment of this subsection and annually thereafter, the Attorney General and the Secretary shall submit to the Committee on the Judiciary of the Senate and the Committee on the Judiciary of the House of Representatives a report regarding the impact of this section, including—

"(A) the number of Federal and State criminal investigations, arrests, indictments, and prosecutions of all cases in which access to ballistics records provided under this section served as a valuable investigative tool in the prosecution of gun crimes;

"(B) the extent to which ballistics records are accessible across jurisdictions; and

"(C) a statistical evaluation of the test programs conducted pursuant to section 6 of the Ballistics, Law Assistance, and State Technology Act.

"(5) There is authorized to be appropriated to the Department of Justice and the Department of the Treasury for each of fiscal years 2001 through 2004, $20,000,000 to carry out this subsection, including—

"(A) installation of ballistics equipment and bullet and cartridge casing recovery equipment;

"(B) establishment of sites for ballistics testing;

"(C) salaries and expenses of necessary personnel; and

"(D) research and evaluation.

"(6) The Secretary and the Attorney General shall conduct mandatory ballistics testing of all firearms obtained or in the possession of their respective agencies."

[Three sections follow dealing with implementation of the act.]

SEC. 5. PRIVACY RIGHTS OF LAW ABIDING CITIZENS.

Ballistics information of individual guns in any form or database established by this Act may not be used for prosecutorial purposes unless law enforcement officials have a reasonable belief that a crime has been committed and that ballistics information would assist in the investigation of that crime.

APPENDIX K

ADVANCING JUSTICE THROUGH DNA TECHNOLOGY (2003)

In 2003, President George W. Bush announced the creation of the President's DNA Initiative. The purpose of the initiative was to find ways of reducing the delay in the use of DNA typing technology in the solving of crimes, in proving the innocence of people improperly accused or convicted of criminal activity, and in the search for missing people. The final report from the National Institute of Justice outlining the objectives and activities of the initiative was called "Advancing Justice through DNA Technology." Some important sections of that report are extracted below.

USING DNA TO SOLVE CRIMES

The past decade has seen great advances in a powerful criminal justice tool: deoxyribonucleic acid, or DNA. DNA can be used to identify criminals with incredible accuracy when biological evidence exists. By the same token, DNA can be used to clear suspects and exonerate persons mistakenly accused or convicted of crimes. In all, DNA technology is increasingly vital to ensuring accuracy and fairness in the criminal justice system.

. . .

DNA is generally used to solve crimes in one of two ways. In cases where a suspect is identified, a sample of that person's DNA can be compared to evidence from the crime scene. The results of this comparison may help establish whether the suspect committed the crime. In cases where a suspect has not yet been identified, biological evidence from the crime scene can be analyzed and compared to offender profiles in DNA databases to help identify the perpetrator. Crime scene evidence can also be linked to other crime scenes through the use of DNA databases.

. . .

Appendix K

DNA evidence is generally linked to DNA offender profiles through DNA databases. In the late 1980s, the federal government laid the groundwork for a system of national, state, and local DNA databases for the storage and exchange of DNA profiles. This system, called the Combined DNA Index System (CODIS), maintains DNA profiles obtained under the federal, state, and local systems in a set of databases that are available to law enforcement agencies across the country for law enforcement purposes. CODIS can compare crime scene evidence to a database of DNA profiles obtained from convicted offenders. CODIS can also link DNA evidence obtained from different crime scenes, thereby identifying serial criminals. . . .

When used to its full potential, DNA evidence will help solve and may even prevent some of the Nation's most serious violent crimes. However, the current federal and state DNA collection and analysis system needs improvement:

(1) In many instances, public crime labs are overwhelmed by backlogs of unanalyzed DNA samples.
(2) In addition, these labs may be ill-equipped to handle the increasing influx of DNA samples and evidence. The problems of backlogs and lack of up-to-date technology result in significant delays in the administration of justice.
(3) More research is needed to develop faster methods for analyzing DNA evidence.
(4) Professionals working in the criminal justice system need additional training and assistance in order to ensure the optimal use of DNA evidence to solve crimes and assist victims.

President Bush believes we must do more to realize the full potential of DNA technology to solve crime and protect the innocent. Under the President's initiative, the Attorney General will improve the use of DNA in the criminal justice system by providing funds and assistance to ensure that this technology reaches its full potential to solve crimes.

1. Eliminating Backlogs

One of the biggest problems facing the criminal justice system today is the substantial backlog of unanalyzed DNA samples and biological evidence from crime scenes, especially in sexual assault and murder cases. Too often, crime scene samples wait unanalyzed in police or crime lab storage facilities. Timely analysis of these samples and placement into DNA databases can avert tragic results. For example, in 1995, the Florida Department of Law Enforcement linked evidence found on a rape-homicide victim to a convicted rapist's DNA profile just eight days before he was scheduled for parole. Had he been released prior to being linked to the unsolved rape-homicide, he may very well have raped or murdered again.

By contrast, analysis and placement into CODIS of DNA profiles can dramatically enhance the chances that potential crime victims will be spared the violence of vicious, repeat offenders. The President's initiative calls for $92.9 million to help alleviate the current backlogs of DNA samples for the most serious violent offenses—rapes, murders, and kidnappings—and for convicted offender samples needing testing. With this additional federal backlog reduction funding, the funding provided by this initiative to improve crime laboratory capacity, and continued support from the states, the current backlogs will be eliminated in five years.

UNDERSTANDING THE BACKLOG

The state and local backlog problem has two components: (1) "casework sample backlogs," which consist of DNA samples obtained from crime scenes, victims, and suspects in criminal cases, and (2) "convicted offender backlogs," which consist of DNA samples obtained from convicted offenders who are incarcerated or under supervision. The nature of the DNA backlog is complex and changing, and measuring the precise number of unanalyzed DNA samples is difficult.

- Casework Sample Backlogs: In a 2001 survey of public DNA laboratories, the Bureau of Justice Statistics (BJS) found that between 1997 and 2000, DNA laboratories experienced a 73% increase in casework and a 135% increase in their casework backlogs. Many casework samples go unanalyzed for lack of a suspect to which to compare the biological evidence from the crime scene. These are often referred to as "no-suspect" cases. Based on an ongoing assessment of crime laboratories and law enforcement agencies, the National Institute of Justice (NIJ) estimates that the current backlog of rape and homicide cases is approximately 350,000. The initiative calls for $76 million in FY 2004 to help eliminate these backlogs over five years.
- Convicted Offender Backlogs: States are increasing the number of convicted offenders required to provide DNA samples. Currently, 23 states require all convicted felons to provide DNA samples. Preliminary estimates by NIJ place the number of collected, untested convicted offender samples at between 200,000 and 300,000. NIJ also estimates that there are between 500,000 and 1,000,000 convicted offender samples that are owed, but not yet collected. The initiative calls for $15 million in FY 2004 to help eliminate convicted offender backlogs over five years.

The federal government also faces a high demand for analysis of casework and convicted offender DNA samples. The FBI has two DNA casework analysis units (see page 5). The first unit, which focuses on analyzing nuclear DNA, has a backlog of approximately 900 cases. The second unit, which focuses on analyzing mitochondrial DNA (mtDNA), has a backlog of roughly 120 cases.

The federal government also collects DNA samples from persons convicted of offenses in certain categories, including crimes of violence or terrorism. The FBI currently has a backlog of approximately 18,000 convicted offender samples. The initiative calls for $1.9 million in FY 2004 to fund the federal convicted offender program; some of these funds will be devoted to eliminating the federal convicted offender backlog.

Effect of Clearing the Backlog

The results of addressing backlogs are dramatic, as the two examples below illustrate:

[Two examples of the use of DNA typing to obtain convictions are given here.]

. . .

Several law enforcement agencies, prosecutors' offices, and crime labs across the country have established innovative programs to review old cases. Often called "cold case units," these programs have enabled criminal justice officials to solve cases that have languished for years without suspects. Most frequently, DNA evidence has been the linchpin in solving these cases. For instance, this past July, a California man was found guilty of the 1974 rape-homicide of a 19-year-old pregnant woman—a case that was solved through DNA evidence nearly thirty years after the crime was committed.

Prior Federal Support of State DNA Backlog Reduction

[This section reviews previous action by the federal government to reduce the backlog of DNA data.]

2. Strengthening Crime Laboratory Capacity

At present, many of our Nation's crime laboratories do not have the capacity necessary to analyze DNA samples in a timely fashion. Many have limited equipment resources, outdated information systems, and overwhelming case management demands. As a result, the criminal justice system as a whole is unable to reap the full benefits of DNA technology. The President's initiative will provide federal funding to further automate and improve the infrastructure of federal, state, and local crime labs so they can process DNA samples efficiently and cost-effectively. These infrastructure improvements are critical to preventing future DNA backlogs, and to helping the criminal justice system realize the full potential of DNA technology.

Increasing the Analysis Capacity of Public Crime Labs

The President's initiative will provide significant support to public crime labs so that these labs can update their infrastructure, automate their DNA analysis procedures, and improve their retention and storage of forensic evidence. The initiative calls for $60 million in FY 2004 funding, which will be dedicated to:

- Providing Basic Infrastructure Support: Some public crime laboratories still need assistance to help them obtain equipment and material to conduct the basic processes of DNA analysis—extraction, quantitation, amplification and analysis—and to help them meet various accreditation requirements.
- Building Infrastructure through Laboratory Information Management Systems: Laboratory Information Management Systems, or "LIMS," are designed to automate evidence handling and casework management, to improve the integrity and speed of evidence handling procedures, and to ensure proper chain of custody. DOJ estimates that only 10 percent of the public DNA laboratories have LIMS systems.
- Providing Automation Tools to Public DNA Laboratories: To streamline aspects of the DNA analysis procedure that are labor and time-intensive, crime laboratories should have automated systems, such as robotic DNA extraction units. Automated DNA analysis systems increase analyst productivity, limit human error and reduce contamination.
- Providing Support for the Retention and Storage of Forensic Evidence: Forensic evidence must be stored in a manner that ensures its integrity and maintains its availability throughout criminal investigations and judicial proceedings. Appropriate evidence storage conditions require costly equipment such as security systems, environmental control systems, ambient temperature monitors, and dehumidifiers. The initiative will support the improvement of evidence storage capabilities.

Funding the FBI Forensic Analysis Programs

The FBI Laboratory runs several different programs for the analysis of DNA information. The Nuclear DNA Program supports federal, state, local, and international law enforcement agencies by providing advanced technical assistance within the forensic biology discipline and subdisciplines through interrelated capabilities and expertise. The Mitochondrial DNA (mtDNA) Analysis Program is responsible for performing mtDNA analysis of forensic evidence containing small or degraded quantities of DNA on items of evidence submitted from federal, state, and local law enforcement agencies. Mitochondrial DNA is a powerful tool available for investigating cases of kidnapping, missing persons, and skeletal remains where nuclear DNA is not present. The initiative will provide funds to these two existing programs to permit them to continue their important work. In addition, the initiative will provide funds to the FBI to further expand regional mtDNA labs that will provide an alternative source for mtDNA analysis to state and local law enforcement, and allow the FBI laboratory to concentrate more of its efforts on federal cases. The initiative calls for $20.5 million in FY 2004 to fund these programs.

Funding the Combined DNA Index System

The Combined DNA Index System (CODIS), administered by the FBI, maintains DNA profiles obtained through federal, state, and local DNA sample collection programs, and makes this information available to law enforcement agencies across the country for law enforcement identification purposes. Currently, the National DNA Index System (NDIS) of CODIS contains about 1.7 million DNA profiles. The President's initiative includes funding to complete a general redesign and upgrade of CODIS, which will increase the system's capacity to 50 million DNA profiles, reduce the search time from hours to microseconds for matching DNA profiles, and enable instant, real-time (as opposed to weekly) searches of the database by participating forensic laboratories. The initiative calls for $9.9 million in FY 2004 to fund this program.

3. Stimulating Research and Development

In order to improve the use of DNA technology to advance the cause of justice, the Attorney General will stimulate research and development of new methods of analyzing DNA samples under the President's initiative. Also, the President has asked the Attorney General to establish demonstration projects under the initiative to further study the public safety and law enforcement benefits of fully integrating the use of DNA technology to solve crimes. Finally, the President has directed the Attorney General to create a National Forensic Science Commission to study rapidly evolving advances in all areas of the forensic sciences and to make recommendations to maximize the use of the forensic sciences in the criminal justice system. In all, the President's initiative will devote $24.8 million in FY 2004 to fund advances in the use of DNA technology.

Improving DNA Technology

Forensic DNA analysis is rapidly evolving. Research and development of tools that will permit crime laboratories to conduct DNA analysis quickly is vital to the goal of improving the timely analysis of DNA samples. Smaller, faster, and less costly analysis tools will reduce capital investments for crime laboratories while increasing their capacity to process more cases. Over the course of the next several years, DNA research efforts will focus on the following areas:

- The development of "DNA chip technology" that uses nanotechnology to improve both speed and resolution of DNA evidence analysis. This technology will reduce analysis time from several hours to several minutes and provide cost-effective miniaturized components.
- The development of more robust methods to enable more crime labs to have greater success in the analysis of degraded, old, or compromised items of biological evidence.
- Advanced applications of various DNA analysis methods, such as automated Short Tandem Repeats (STRs), Single Nucleotide Polymorphisms (SNPs), mitochondrial DNA analysis (mtDNA), and Y-chromosome DNA analysis.
- The use of animal, plant, and microbial DNA to provide leads that may link DNA found on or near human perpetrators or victims to the actual perpetrator of the crime.
- Technologies that will enable DNA identification of vast numbers of samples occasioned by a mass disaster or mass fatality incident.
- Technologies that permit better separation of minute traces of male sexual assailant DNA from female victims.

The initiative devotes $10 million in FY 2004 funding to benefit the state and local criminal justice community through DNA research and development. It also requests $9.8 million in FY 2004 funding to further expand the FBI's DNA research and development program.

Establishing DNA Demonstration Projects

[This section describes demonstration projects that will be supported by the initiative.]

Creating a National Forensic Science Commission

To facilitate the ability of policymakers to assess the needs of the forensic science community, and to stimulate public awareness of the uses of forensic technology to solve crimes, the President has directed the Attorney General to create a National Forensic Science Commission. The Commission will be charged with two primary responsibilities: (1) developing recommendations for long-term strategies to maximize the use of current forensic technologies to solve crimes and protect the public, and (2) identifying potential scientific breakthroughs that may be used to assist law enforcement.

The Attorney General will appoint Commission members from professional forensic science organizations and accreditation bodies and from the criminal justice community. These individuals will have broad knowledge and in-depth expertise in the criminal justice system and in various areas of the forensic sciences such as analytical toxicology, trace evidence, forensic biology, firearms and toolmark examinations, latent fingerprints, crime scene analysis, digital evidence, and forensic pathology, in addition to DNA. Judges, prosecutors, attorneys, victim advocates, and other members of the criminal justice system will also be represented on the Commission.

The Commission will study advances in all areas of the forensic sciences and make recommendations on how new and existing technologies can be used to improve public safety. The Commission will also serve as an ongoing forum for discussing initiatives and policy, and may issue recommendations that will assist state and local law enforcement agencies in the cost-effective use of these technologies to solve crimes. The initiative devotes $500,000 in FY 2004 to the establishment of the Commission.

4. Training the Criminal Justice Community

In order to maximize the use of DNA technology, under the President's initiative, the Attorney General will develop training and provide assistance regarding the collection and use of DNA evidence to the wide variety of professionals involved in the criminal justice system, including police officers, prosecutors, defense attorneys, judges, forensic scientists, medical personnel, victim service providers, corrections officers, and probation and parole officers.

Key players in the criminal justice system should receive additional training in the proper collection, preservation, and use of DNA evidence. Fundamental knowledge of the capabilities of DNA technology is essential for police officers to collect evidence properly, prosecutors and defense attorneys to introduce and use it successfully in court, and judges to rule correctly on its admissibility. Victim service providers and medical personnel likewise need to understand DNA technology in order to encourage more successful evidence collection and to be fully responsive to the needs of victims.

Law Enforcement Training

As the first responders to crime scenes, law enforcement officers should be able to identify, collect and preserve probative biological evidence for submission to crime laboratories. Improper collection can mean that valuable evidence is missed or rendered unsuitable for testing. The initiative devotes $3.5 million in FY 2004 to assist law enforcement in meeting the following training needs:

- Basic "awareness training" on DNA evidence for patrol officers and other first-responders;
- Intensive training on identifying, collecting, and preserving potential DNA evidence for evidence technicians, investigators, and others processing crime scenes;
- Training and education for investigators and responding officers on DNA databases and their potential to provide leads in current and "cold" cases; and
- Training and information for law enforcement leadership and policymakers to facilitate more informed decisions about effective DNA evidence collection and testing.

[The rest of this section provides details of plans for the training of prosecutors, defense attorneys, and judges; probation and parole officers and corrections personnel; forensic scientists; medical personnel; and victim service providers.

. . .

USING DNA TO PROTECT THE INNOCENT

DNA technology is increasingly vital to ensuring fairness in the criminal justice system. Every effort that is made to reduce backlogs of untested evidence, to better equip forensic laboratories, to develop faster methods of analyzing samples, and to better train professionals in the use of DNA technology, will improve the accuracy of the criminal justice system. Accordingly, the measures described in the previous sections will not only help solve crimes and keep dangerous offenders off the streets, but will also help minimize the risk that innocent individuals are wrongly accused or convicted.

. . .

[The section continues with two examples in which DNA testing was used to exonerate individuals convicted of crimes.]

. . .

Many states have already enacted provisions that allow convicted offenders in certain cases to seek post-conviction DNA testing of evidence collected in those cases. Currently, 31 states have enacted special statutory provisions providing post-conviction DNA testing, and additional states make post-conviction testing available through other procedures. Federal law also should provide for post-conviction DNA testing in appropriate cases.

To demonstrate support for appropriate post-conviction testing of DNA evidence, the Attorney General will create a $5 million grant program under the President's initiative to help states defray the costs of post-conviction DNA testing. In order to receive this funding, state programs will be required to meet criteria established by the Department of Justice. These criteria will require that DNA testing be performed by an accredited forensic laboratory, and will encourage states to develop plans that ensure prompt DNA testing of persons who may be wrongly convicted and discourage frivolous testing that may cause unnecessary expense and needless harm to crime victims.

USING DNA TO IDENTIFY MISSING PERSONS

Families of missing persons who are presumed dead face tremendous emotional turmoil when they are unable to learn about the fates of their loved ones. The events of September 11, 2001 demonstrated on a national scale the potential for anguish when the remains of a missing person go unidentified. In the wake of this tragedy, the Department of Justice brought together DNA experts from across the country to develop improved DNA analysis methods identifying the World Trade Center victims.

Despite tremendous scientific advancements, DNA technology is not routinely used in missing persons cases. According to statistics maintained by the FBI's National Crime Information Center (NCIC), there are nearly 5,000 reported unidentified persons in the United States. This element of the President's initiative will help identify the missing, and in doing so, will provide an increased sense of closure to their families.

The FBI's Missing Persons DNA Database Program currently provides the essential infrastructure for identifying human remains. This database maintains two indices of DNA samples. The first index contains DNA profiles of relatives of missing persons and the second contains DNA profiles of unidentified human remains. Successful identifications require that both profiles be entered. Currently, this database is not used to its full potential. States have only recently begun to conduct DNA analysis on human remains and to submit the results to the FBI for inclusion in its database. Many unidentified human remains continue to be disposed of without the collection of DNA samples. Further, even when the samples are collected, many crime labs lack the capacity to conduct timely analysis, especially where the biological sample is old or degraded. In addition, many family members and law enforcement officials lack sufficient information about the existence of the program and how to participate.

The President's initiative will help ensure that DNA forensic technology is used to its full potential to identify missing persons. The initiative will:

- Provide outreach and education to medical examiners, coroners, and law enforcement officers about the use of DNA to identify human remains and to aid in missing persons cases;
- Make DNA reference collection kits available to these state and local officials;
- Support the development of educational materials and outreach programs for families of missing children and adults;
- Encourage states to collect DNA samples before any unidentified remains are disposed;
- Strengthen crime lab capacity (see page 4) to enable more state and local labs to conduct timely DNA analysis of biological samples from unidentified human remains;
- Provide for the analysis of degraded and old biological samples through the FBI's Mitochondrial DNA Analysis Program (see page 5);
- Provide technical assistance to state and local crime labs and medical examiners on the collection and analysis of degraded remains through the FBI and the National Institute of Justice; and
- Support research and development of more robust methods for analyzing degraded, old, or compromised biological samples (see page 6).

The President's initiative will devote $2 million in FY 2004 for outreach programs and the development of educational materials and reference collection kits.

INDEX

Locators in **boldface** indicate main topics. Locators followed by *c* indicate chronology entries. Locators followed by *b* indicate biographical entries. Locators followed by *g* indicate glossary entries.

Index

Index

Index

Index

Index

Index

Index